FOUNDERS

FOUNDERS

C. MAX LANG

David E. Jenkins, Jr., John A. Waldhausen, Editors

Library of Congress Control Number:		2015907485
ISBN:	Hardcover	978-1-5035-6952-2
	Softcover	978-1-5035-6951-5
	eBook	978-1-5035-6950-8

Print information available on the last page.

Rev. date: 05/14/2015

To order additional copies of this book, contact:
Xlibris
1-888-795-4274
www.Xlibris.com
Orders@Xlibris.com
714333

Contents

Dedication

To the memory of George T. Harrell, M.D., founding Dean, College of Medicine, Senior Vice President of The Milton S. Hershey Medical Center of The Pennsylvania State University. It was his vision that inspired us to achieve our goals.

Acknowledgements

Melvin "Bub" Parker, University Development and Alumni Affairs, TMSHMC

Xuwen Peng, DVM, MS, PhD, Associate Professor, Department of Comparative Medicine, TMSHMC

Mrs Bonnie C. Whalen, Administrative Research Resource Specialist, Department of Comparative Medicine, TMSHMC

Ms Atrya Reigle, Administrative Support Assistant, Department of Comparative Medicine, TMSHMC

Ms Ester Dell, Associate Librarian, ILL/Reference, George T. Harrell Library, TMSHMC

Ms Eileen R. Wiley, Asst Dir, Facilities Planning and Construction, TMSHMC

Dr Cheston Berlin, Kenneth L. Miller, and Dr Elliot Vesell for their insight and editorial review of the manuscript.

Significant financial support was provided by

David E. Jenkins

C. Max Lang

John A. Waldhausen

Marketing, TMSHMC

Office of Faculty Development, TMSHMC

University Development, TMSHMC

Royalties from this book will be donated to The Penn State College of Medicine Alumni Society Scholarship Fund

PREFACE

The founding of The Milton S. Hershey Medical Center was described in *The Impossible Dream, C. Max Lang, AuthorHouse, 2010; 1663 Liberty Drive, Bloomington, IN 47403; www.authorhouse. com*. Its focus was the people and events that resulted in the accumulation of funds ($50 million in 1963; $388 million in 2014 dollars) to build a new medical school approximately 90 miles from the parent university (The Pennsylvania State University). Background material for that book is in Appendix 4.

After publication of *The Impossible Dream*, which covered the period mid 1950's to 1966, there were many suggestions to write another book on the founders of this new medical school, emphasizing their vision and goals. Drs. C. Max Lang, David E. Jenkins, Jr. and John A. Waldhausen agreed to undertake this task. Unfortunately, Dr. Waldhausen passed away in 2012, leaving Drs. Lang and Jenkins to complete this history of our institution for the period 1967 to 1987. A lapse of 25 or more years was believed appropriate to assess the impact of activities.

The focus of the present book is to examine the role of the senior leaders, department chairs, division chiefs, senior faculty, and administrators involved in this venture with a focus on their vision and goals and, upon reflection, their achievements. The information is based on their curriculum vitae, oral interviews (recorded, using a standardized format for consistency), information from the files, and personal recollections. Their curriculum vitae (at time of interview) and interview transcripts are available electronically (Appendices 1 and 2).

CHAPTER 1

BACKGROUND

Medical education has evolved over centuries. It most likely started with clergy who, by their calling, provided compassionate care to their flock. As time progressed, they began to experiment with herbs and other substances. This, in turn, required additional help to prepare these substances. Perhaps this was the beginning of "medical education". This informal instruction continued until the 19th century when others saw the opportunity to make money by selling remedies and offering "consultation". By the late 1800's Americans were becoming very upset about the inadequate level of medical care, especially the lack of knowledge and medical training. In fact, by the early 1900's, 90% of the "doctors" had never been to college, let alone a "proper medical school." This led to a series of cascading events that, eventually, led to the type of medical education that we have today and continues to evolve. The seminal events were the Flexner report, World War II and NIH,

The Flexner Report (Flexner, A, 1910, *Medical Education in the United States and Canada: A Report to the Carnegie Foundation for the Advancement of Teaching.* Bulletin No 4, New York City) reiterated the frustrations of the American public pertaining to the delivery of adequate medical care, deficiencies in medical education, and failure of the government to provide some oversight. The reaction to this report was swift, but not complete. State laws were enacted setting the standards for medical education and licensure. However, many of the "doctors" were grandfathered under these new rules and remained in practice; most of the "trade" medical schools closed but many of the drug stores continued to have a "medical school" in a back room. The "students" learned their trade by making medicines from herbs and other compounds (alcohol being a common ingredient) and observation of their mentor. It is interesting that almost all doctors advertised themselves as "Physicians and Surgeons" until the mid-1950's.

In the early 1900's, the standards for medical education were formalized but the faculty consisted, primarily, of physicians in private practice especially for the clinical training. This arrangement of part time faculty was not ideal; transportation between the hospital and practice site, coordination of student and mentor schedules, and student participation frequently interrupted the physician's schedule and, in turn, his/her income. As a result, most of the clinical teaching was in the hospital—with the patient in a horizontal position, a small portion of patient care compared to overall patient treatment.

Dr. Harrell, founding Dean of the College of Medicine, TPSU became a physician during this era. He was the first clinical faculty member of the Bowman Gray School of Medicine (BGSM now Wake Forest University or WFU) which was transitioning from a 2 year (preclinical) to a 4 year medical school (preclinical and clinical). He did receive a very modest faculty salary, but the bulk of his income was derived from seeing private patients in the hospital.

The advent of World War II was the next major impact on medical education. The military's experience with World War I made the government acutely aware that the United States simply did not have the medical resources to meet the needs of the civilian population and the military. This resulted in several changes: dramatic increases in medical school class size; some decrease in the length of medical school; admission to medical school with minimal or no previous college experience; and sending military draftees to medical school based on aptitude tests. All of these changes put a tremendous strain on the medical schools, with an increase in the number of faculty, both full time and part time, including basic and clinical sciences.

As World War II drew to a close, *bona fide* medical schools in the United States had a large faculty but fewer students, increased research space that had been built to address military issues, and many faculty who had developed a strong interest in research. This impetus, plus a shifting of national economics, led to the establishment and an expansion of the National Institutes of Health (NIH). These factors enabled the Federal government to fund new, additional research and medical education facilities and investigator-initiated research. All of these events had a positive impact on medical education, e.g., more faculty, thus increasing the time for student/faculty interaction; new knowledge from both basic and clinical science research; and advances in technology, improving basic science research and patient care. However, on the basis of like begets like, most of the clinical faculty had been trained in the part time/private practice modem continuing the problem of faculty availability and institutional loyalty.

The gradual change from part time to full time faculty has had a positive influence on medical education; however that trend is now reversing, especially in the clinical sciences because faculty salaries are often based on patient fees, and at the expense of time for teaching and research. Most of the basic science faculty are full time and some departments have dramatically increased in size. This was made possible, primarily, because of research funding. However, the steady decline in research funding raises the question of sustainability. Many of these faculty have tenure, making it difficult to correct the problem—especially for those faculty who are relatively unproductive in teaching/research. This problem can only be resolved by stronger department leadership and a change in the tenure concept.

CHAPTER 2

LEADERSHIP

Leadership at The Milton S. Hershey Medical Center (TMSHMC) varied since its inception; perhaps such variation has been most notable at the level of the President of The Pennsylvania State University (TPSU), and somewhat at the level of the Dean of the College of Medicine. There has been little change with the department chairs (in the period covered by this book, i.e. 1967-87), primarily, because there was little turnover in the first 30 years.

The first duo, President Eric A. Walker and Dean George T. Harrell, was superb. They had full confidence in each other and saw a common goal; even though President Walker failed to have part, or all, of TMSHMC at University Park PA (the location of the main University campus) because of the legal stipulations associated with the gift of $50 million from the Hershey Trust Company in 1963. Dean Harrell established the initial goals and a vision for this new school; which was transferred to/and readily accepted by the founding chairs.

President Walker was succeeded by John W. Oswald, and that mutual respect between the President and Dean ceased to exist. President Oswald handled the transition of the College of Medicine Deans rather poorly and rumors among the faculty ran rampant until President Oswald met with the Executive Committee (composed of the academic department chairs) and made the announcement of a change in leadership of the Dean of the College of Medicine. Dean Harrell was only one year from mandatory retirement and Dr. John A. Waldhausen (Chair of Surgery) was chosen by President Oswald to be the Interim Provost & Dean (1972-73) and mutual respect was restored. Dr. Harrell was appointed Vice President for Health Affairs for his final year before mandatory retirement. Waldhausen was reluctant to accept the responsibility because he was still building his department of Surgery and felt a strong sense of obligation to his young faculty. Finally, he agreed to accept the position subject to the following requirements for TMSHMC: (1) develop an independent Personnel Department to deal with all employment at the Hershey Medical Center; (2) develop an independent Grants and Contracts Office; and (3) have more competitive salaries. Personnel issues had been a constant problem with University Park not understanding the issues that were developing at the medical center. Grant and Contract applications were increasing, especially to the NIH, and the distance between Hershey and University Park was a major problem in the application review process. The Sponsored Research Office at University Park was excellent in dealing with most government funding programs, but had little experience with the NIH.

To the relief of the faculty, Dr. Waldhausen decided that he would not change the trajectory of the institution's mission. President Oswald asked Dr. Waldhausen to be the permanent Dean but he declined because, again, he was still building his department and felt an obligation to his young faculty. Waldhausen and Oswald had an excellent working relationship and mutual respect. It is interesting to note that after Oswald appointed a permanent Dean (Prystowsky), he did not seek advice or input from Waldhausen. Thus, the pattern was emerging that each President selects his own Dean.

President Oswald recruited Dr. Harry Prystowsky from the University of Florida to succeed Dr. Waldhausen as Vice President for Health Affairs and Dean of the College of Medicine. Prystowsky and Oswald clearly worked hand in hand. TMSHMC was heavily in debt when Prystowsky was appointed, primarily due to the start-up costs of the new hospital; many expenses and little income. Drs. Harrell and Waldhausen understood that such was inevitable and would correct itself in time. President Walker also understood this—he even projected this loss to the Hershey Foundation, even before construction was started, to be in the range of $25 million. However, the University Trustees did not understand, and many were poised to close the yet to be built medical center and return the money to the Hershey Foundation. In fact, when Dr. Prystowsky was presented to the Board of Trustees, there were two potential motions to be made: (1) appoint Prystowsky as Vice President for Health Affairs and Dean of the College of Medicine with the understanding that he would resolve the financial issues, and (2) close TMSHMC and return the $50 million to the Hershey Foundation. The second motion was never made. An interesting anecdote was when Dr. Waldhausen and a colleague, looking out the hospital window at a relatively empty parking lot, suggested that we haul in a bunch of junked cars so it would look like we were busy and stimulate more admissions. Nevertheless, Dr. Prystowsky was given the primary charge of putting TMSHMC on sound financial footing; and he did so in a superb manner. Some thought that he excelled more in his position as Chair of the Department of Obstetrics and Gynecology at the University of Florida than as Dean of TMSHMC. I (CML) disagree; both required goals, vision, and vigor—it was only the focus that was different. Since his focus was on finances, he retained the goals and vision of Harrell and Waldhausen; primarily by empowering the department chairs in subtle and not so subtle ways. One of his first acts was to put pictures of all of the department chairs on the wall of the Executive Conference Room (he later had portraits of all of the chairs hung in the hospital auditorium). The unspoken message was "these are the members of my team and I have full confidence in their abilities". Subsequent deans removed the pictures and portraits, sending a different message.

Dr. Oswald was succeeded by Dr. Bryce Jordan who was trained in the arts and had little understanding of science. He tried, repeatedly, to tap the medical center finances which, by then, had improved significantly. Obviously, Jordan and Prystowsky did not see eye to eye, and Dr. Prystowsky decided to take early retirement; he had accomplished all of his personal and professional goals.

CHAPTER 3

RECRUITMENT OF FACULTY TO THE MILTON S. HERSHEY MEDICAL CENTER (TMSHMC) OF THE PENNSYLVANIA STATE UNIVERSITY (TPSU)

Dr. George T. Harrell, founding Dean, established the criteria for department chairs: teaching expertise; research productivity, and, in the case of clinical faculty, superb patient care; personal interactions and leadership skills; and age. He strongly believed that education is the primary goal of an academic medical center; in fact, he strongly supported the concept that the word "doctor" comes from the Latin word "to teach". He was looking for individuals who had a track record of excellent, innovative teaching. He considered research to be an integral part of teaching, providing new information to our existing body of knowledge; and demonstrating problem solving skills to the students. He was not so interested in the subject of research (as long as it was relevant to the discipline) or the number of publications. The publications had to be in good journals and the data "accurate to the last millimeter." Age, in terms of years, is probably a misnomer. Dr. Harrell, as a medical student, noticed that the younger faculty at Duke University were more enthusiastic and willing to try innovative approaches to educating the students. He did not want to recruit people who were already chairs, or even a vice chair, because he thought they would just repeat what they had been doing rather than being innovative. He used that approach when he was Dean of the College of Medicine at the University of Florida prior to his coming to TMSHMC and thought that it was very successful.

Several Chairs and Division Chiefs had previous military experience. This was probably a reflection of the time, i.e. World War II, Korea, and Viet Nam. Some were drafted, and sent to medical school on the basis of an aptitude test; others volunteered under the Berry Plan (could interrupt residency training and most would be guaranteed a place in the residency program upon completion of their military service); some continued their education under the GI Bill; and others volunteered because they knew that they would be drafted. Nevertheless, serving in the uniform services did appear to have beneficial effects; leadership skills, following orders, and for some a career decision not previously considered.

Department Chairs	Division Chiefs		Administrators
Lang, USA	Abt, USPHS	Ladda, USA	Bryant, USA
Leaman, T, USA	Bardin, USPHS	Leaman, D, USPHS	Corley, USA
Morgan, USA	Berlin, USPHS	Maisels, USA	Russell, USA
Munger, USAF	Conner, USN	Muller, USAF	
Nelson, USA	Demers, USA	Nahrwold, USA	
Pattishall, USN	DeMuth, USA	Page, USN	
Vastyan, USAF	Dossett, USAF	Pierce, USPHS	
Vesell, USPHS	Greer, USA	Santen, USPHS	
Waldhausen, USPHS	Hayes, USA	Severs, USA	
Weidner, USN	Houts, USA	Zelis, USPHS	
Yeakel. USN	Krieg, USAF		

Dr. Harrell had a unique advantage in recruiting. When he accepted the Deanship at Florida, the President of the University suggested that Harrell and the architect visit all of the medical schools built or significantly expanded since World War II. Dr. Harrell was a frequent lecturer at national medical meetings, and served on several national committees on medical education and construction of medical and patient care facilities. Accordingly, he was well known, and aware of who had outstanding programs. He contacted individuals, using this knowledge, and sought suggestions of potential outstanding candidates. He then asked these candidates to come for an interview, usually with their spouse because he knew their important role in this new venture. Although Dr. Harrell was the primary recruiter, he did ask those chairs who were on board to interview all of the candidates and give him their recommendations.

Dr. Harrell's recruiting was national in scope because of his contacts, but most Chairs recruited from people that they had worked with at previous appointments. Founding chairs were generally distinguished scholars, collegial, interactive, and supportive of each other. Most appointed Chairs had not previously been above the rank of Associate Professor or had any prior significant administrative experience. Thus, they had to lean on each other. Another attribute was that they felt comfortable in critiquing each other without hard feelings; just gratitude for helpful advice. All of them were attracted by the opportunity to build the best departments possible in any entirely new medical school and setting. To accomplish this, they were amazingly free to innovate and unrestrained. The former traditions and restrictions that prevailed in older institutions where they had been trained and/or served as faculty members simply did not apply to TMSHMC—a unique chance to make their dreams come true.

CHAPTER 4

FUNDING

Initially, TMSHMC received no funding from the Commonwealth of Pennsylvania; operating costs were from the Hershey Foundation gift, and limited University funds. Thus, the faculty salaries, number of academic departments, and number of faculty per department were dictated by the Hershey Foundation and the University. Mr. Hinkle, representing the Hershey Foundation, recommended that the Dean's salary be in the range of $30-35,000, preferably at the lower end. Harrell's starting salary was $30,000 ($233,188 in 2014 adjusted for inflation). He did not receive a pay increase during his first 3 years as Dean, and he retired at an annual salary of $40,800. It was often thought that this salary level may have reflected that of the various Hershey executives. President Walker readily agreed with this salary for Dr. Harrell, because he was concerned about any significant salary disparity between faculty in the College of Medicine and faculty elsewhere in the University. Based on the Dean's salary, this automatically set the salaries in the range of $20,000 for Basic Science Chairs and $25,000 for Clinical Science Chairs ($146,822 and $183,528, respectively in 2014 adjusted for inflation). These salary ranges were low in comparison to other medical schools, and Dr. Harrell was able to get a few exceptions; however it is believed that none, or most, individuals did not receive any more than what they were already making at their previous institution at the time of their appointment. The ultimate salary range, at the time of appointment, was $13,428-27,500 for Basic Science Chairs and $29,000-42,000 for Clinical Science Chairs. Dr. Harrell was reluctant to discuss salaries with the Chair candidates, and even his own with the President. This was probably due, in part, to the fact that he did not have the final authority; that resided with the Hershey Foundation and the President of the University.

The number of academic departments was established by Dr. Harrell, subject to the approval of the Hershey Foundation and the University President. Basic Science departments are involved in teaching and research, whereas the Clinical Science departments are also involved in patient care. The initial Academic Departments were:

Basic Science	Clinical Science
Anatomy	Anesthesiology
Behavioral Science	Family & Community Medicine
Biological Chemistry	Medicine
Comparative Medicine	Obstetrics & Gynecology
Humanities	Pathology
Microbiology	Pediatrics
Pharmacology	Psychiatry
Physiology	Radiology
	Surgery

In subsequent years, Anatomy was merged with Behavioral Science and re-named, first to Neuroscience & Anatomy, then Neural and Behavioral Sciences; the name of Biological Chemistry was changed to Biological Chemistry & Molecular Biology; and Physiology was changed to Cellular and Molecular Physiology. Previous divisions were formed as separate departments from initial departments: Neurosurgery, Ophthalmology and Orthopedic Surgery from Surgery, and Dermatology and Neurology from Medicine, and a new Department of Health Evaluation Sciences. The change in the names of the Basic Science departments was made to better indicate their teaching and research programs, and to communicate the same to prospective graduate students and postdoctoral fellows. The new departments in the Clinical Sciences reflected growth and what was perceived to be manageable.

As the College of Medicine grew (class size, research programs, and patient care), the original allotment of the number of faculty was clearly inadequate; however, it was at a time when the TMSHMC deficit was growing, mainly due to start-up costs of the Teaching Hospital. Basic Science departments were initially allotted 5 faculty members except for Humanities which was 3, and Comparative Medicine had 1. The solution was the development of the Interim Research Pool (IRP) and Academic Enrichment Fund (AEF). The IRP was generated from salary savings of tenured/tenure eligible faculty from research/contract funds and gifts. These moneys could be used to hire additional non-tenure faculty and technicians, equipment or other items to meet the education and research needs of the department. The rules were quite flexible and under the control of the Chair. The AEF was operated in much the same manner but was derived mainly from clinical income. Some departments, both Basic Science and Clinical Science, returned the money to the investigators to expand their research programs, some shared the money with the investigator, and the rest to meet departmental needs. Others used the funds as they saw fit. Any change in these formulae will have a significant impact on the institution's future growth and development.

CHAPTER 5

BASIC SCIENCE ACADEMIC DEPARTMENTS

DEPARTMENT of ANATOMY – BRYCE L(eon) MUNGER, M.D., founding Chair, 1966-91. He was born May 20, 1933 in Everett, WA (died October,15, 2004). He graduated from Everett High School in 1951 as *Salutatorian*, and was known as a student leader. He attended the University of Washington and received Faculty Medalist Awards in 1953 and 1954 for having the highest grades of 4,000 students. He was elected to Phi Beta Kappa in 1953. He was an accomplished concert pianist and had to make the difficult decision of a career; music or medicine. He chose the latter and was admitted to Washington University, St Louis, MO in 1954, after 3 years of undergraduate education. As a medical student, he was elected to Alpha Omega Alpha (1957) and Society of Sigma Xi (1957) and received the Borden (1958) and Roche (1958) Awards for academic excellence; and graduated in 1958, *summa cum laude*.

Munger was an Intern in Pathology and Assistant in Pathology at The Johns Hopkins University Hospital, 1958- 59. Because of the military draft (Berry Plan), he entered the United States Air Force (USAF) as a Captain and served as Investigator in Experimental Pathology, The Armed Forces Institute of Pathology, 1959-61. During that time, he established an Electron Microscopy Laboratory as a resource for experimental pathology.

Munger's goal was to be a Department Chair in a medical school, although his primary goal was to do research. He received several offers for a faculty appointment and chose the institution that he believed offered the best opportunity to ultimately become a Chair. He started his academic career as an Assistant Professor of Anatomy, Washington University (1961-65), then Associate Professor of Anatomy, The University of Chicago, School of Medicine (1965-66).

He was appointed Professor and Chairman of Anatomy, College of Medicine, TPSU in 1966. He and his wife, Donna, decided to drive for the interview; first to University Park to meet with President Walker, and then to Hershey. At that time, all faculty to be appointed as a Professor had to be interviewed by the President, and those to make over $20,000/year by the Hershey Foundation.

After his appointment as Professor and Chairman, Department of Anatomy, TMSHMC, TPSU (1966-87), he remained on the faculty as Professor of Neuroscience and Anatomy, TMSHMC, TPSU (1988-91). He then served as Professor and Head, Department of Anatomy, University of Tasmania, Hobart, Tasmania, Australia (1992-1996), then as Professor of Anatomy and Physiology (1996-97); he concurrently served as Assistant Dean for Student Affairs, Pre-clinical (1993-97) at the same University. He later served as Visiting Professor of Cell Biology, Neurobiology and Anatomy, Ohio State University, Columbus, OH (Fall, 1997) and Adjunct Professor of Anatomy, Midwestern University, Arizona College of Osteopathic Medicine, Glendale Campus, Phoenix, AZ (1999-2000).

Munger's vision was to develop a research oriented department with an emphasis on education. He approached the development of his department with vigor and enthusiasm. His first act was to hire a remarkable histotechnician, Ms Eileen Sevier, to prepare histology slides in what had formerly been a kitchen in a home for the Milton Hershey students, using rat tissues, for the incoming class of 40 medical students. She made many more sets than required in case of breakage and future increases in class size. Munger reviewed every slide to ensure that they were up to his standards—and they were! A graduate student (Dennis Stanton) of Dr. Munger accompanied him from the University of Chicago to finish his PhD thesis project.

His project involved the dissection of embalmed monkeys, and the formalin smell was too overwhelming to share the kitchen, and the rest of the building, so he used the milk house at Gro-Mor barn as his dissecting laboratory; becoming the first research laboratory at TMSHMC; and people today are so picky about their laboratories!

His first recruit was Irwin Baird, PhD, to teach Gross Anatomy, and he was superb. He also recruited Drs. Ben (PhD) and Lillian Pubols (PhD), a husband-wife team, who transferred from the College of Science at University Park. They, too, were enthusiastic about teaching. They followed up on Munger's earlier work with the raccoon and studied the mechanoreceptors in its' forepaw. It was a commonly held belief that raccoons washed their food for cleansing. However, the Pubols showed that the action of washing the food in water was to increase the sensitivity of their fingers and, in turn, decide whether the substance was edible. A later recruit was Ian Zagon, Ph.D. Zagon gradually took over the teaching of Gross Anatomy and routinely received the Distinguished Teacher of The Year Award from the first year medical students. He is also a very productive investigator studying the effects of opioids and has received several million dollars in peer reviewed research grants, resulting in more than 200 publications in peer-reviewed journals

Munger, himself, was a very productive investigator, studying mechanoreceptors and cytopathology in skin and organs in a variety of animals, including rabbits, rats, monkeys, raccoons, opossums, guinea pigs, and snakes, and published 119 peer reviewed papers. Snakes have a very primitive pancreas, in terms of cellular structure, and posed some interesting requirements in their care and handling. Some of the species were called "one step" snakes because that is as far as one could go after being bitten and before passing out. This, of course, required a few precautionary measures, e.g. keeping the anti-venoms on hand, no entry into the room unless another person was observing through the door window, and the investigator/technician carrying an open umbrella to ward off the striking fangs.

Munger was among the first to describe "delta" cells in the pancreas which are new islet cells resulting from insulin deficiency and increased blood glucose. These cells are rarely seen in diabetic humans because of insulin administration to avoid ketosis and, in turn, death. However, they do occur in severely diabetic guinea pigs which do not develop diabetic ketosis—despite the fact that guinea pigs frequently develop pregnancy ketosis. Munger was honored by the Japan Society for the Promotion of Science Fellowship (1987) and the Purkinje Medal, Czechoslovakia (1987).

He maintained his interest in music, and organized The Hershey Symphony Orchestra, serving as its first Director and Conductor.

Munger was the moving force behind the initiation, and subsequent passage, of the Organ and Tissue Donation Law of Pennsylvania. This law has been used as a model by other states.

Munger's wife, Donna, was also a distinguished professional historian and geneologist. She completed the requirements for a PhD in history, and is perhaps best known for her publications on *Connecticut's Pennsylvania "Colony" 1754-1810. Susquehanna Company Proprietors, Settlers, and Claimants*. Similar to her husband, she approached everything with vigor and enthusiasm.

DEPARTMENT of BEHAVIORAL SCIENCE – EVAN G(radick) PATTISHALL, Jr, Ph.D., M.D., founding chair, 1966-80. Pattishall was born in Richmond, VA, September 2, 1921 (died July 8, 2003). He started college at Davidson College (1939-41). His college education was interrupted by military service; he served as a Lieutenant in the United States Naval Reserve, 1943-48, (Amphibious Fleet, South Pacific). After his military service, he continued his education at the University of Michigan receiving a B.M. (1947), and M.M. (1948), and a Ph.D. (1951, Educational Psychology). He spent a year at Appalachian State College as an Assistant Professor of Psychology (1950-51). He then worked for the Office of Naval Research as a Research Psychologist (1951-53). He was appointed to the faculty of the University of Virginia as an Assistant Professor of Psychology (1953-54), plus Educational Research (1954-56), then promoted to Associate Professor in 1956. He also served as Director of the Division of Educational Research (1955-58). He left Virginia to attend medical school at the Western Reserve University (WRU) Cleveland, OH, receiving his M.D. in 1962.

Pattishall's first medical school appointment was at the University of Florida as Associate Professor and Chief of the Division of Behavioral Sciences, Department of Psychiatry (1962-66). He served concurrently as Chair of the Medical Student Admissions Committee.

He was appointed as Professor and Chair of the Department of Behavioral Science at Hershey in 1966; the first Department of this type in a medical school, reflecting Dr. Harrell's goal that he first envisioned in the 1930's but was unable to accomplish at BGSM/WFU and could only partially accomplish, by subterfuge, at the University of Florida. Pattishall also served as the Head of the Medical School Selection Committee; Dr. Harrell was adamant that it not be called Admissions Committee.

Pattishall's vision and goals were less clear; he was strongly interested in being a department chair and in medical education; and his earlier career suggests searching for a niche. His early publications reflected his interest in educational psychology. Dr. Harrell's vision was that the students should learn normal behavior before they learned abnormal behavior, i. e. Psychiatry, and, based on his experience as a *loco tenens* while still a resident in medicine, where he realized that many patients had no organic illness but only behavioral manifestations or behavioral overtones. Pattishall approached his vision by recruiting a pediatric psychiatrist (Offord), a social scientist (Houts), and an animal behavioralist (Thompson). Dan Offord, M.D., was very good but he ran a youth camp in Canada for troubled teens (he was a Canadian citizen) which was his primary interest. Peter Houts, Ph.D., was also a very good teacher and a confidant of Pattishall, and they had many discussions about the vision and goals of the department; he had many excellent suggestions, but it appeared that Pattishall could never "quite get his arms around the concepts" in order to develop a clear focus and develop a definitive curriculum. Carl Thompson, PhD was clearly out of his league. He did his postgraduate work with nonhuman primates in one of the NIH supported Primate Centers. He was well trained for that work, and continued his studies at TMSHMC on left handedness in monkeys. However, he felt isolated and left after a few years to teach psychology at a small, liberal arts college in the Midwest.

PETER S(teven) HOUTS, Ph.D. (Social Psychology) was dedicated to patients and their families, including the study of economic and psychological burdens of the disease to improving the quality of life for patients with cancer. He studied different aspects of how illness, especially cancer, and its effects on patients and their families, including the economic and psychological burdens of disease, and the effect of treatments on the quality of life. He is well known for his teaching and research. He studied, and published, the behavioral impact of the Three Mile Island Nuclear Accident which occurred in 1979, just 8 ½ miles from TMSHMC. Publications included topics on evacuation, economic impacts, stress, and attitudes.

As a result and/or combination of his life experiences and education in social psychology he had a very unique insight in many areas. His research lead to many innovations and programs around the country. All of these factors gave him a good perspective on medical school curricula.

After Houts retired in 1998, he attended art school for three years, where he studied graphic design. During that time, the digital camera was introduced. And, he began to learn digital photography. His subjects expanded from people in family portraits to the outdoors when in 2004, he began to photograph Hershey Gardens for a book about its history (*Hershey Gardens: The Cornfield that Blossomed with Roses*), written in conjunction with his wife, Mary Davidoff Houts.

JANICE A. EGELAND, Ph.D. (Medical Behavioral Science – Commonwealth Fund Fellow, (Yale) (AB/Microbiology – Phi Beta Kappa junior year, Penn); MA (Sociology – Medical, Penn). Egeland was the 4th faculty appointment (Lang, Pattishall, Munger preceded her) in 1967. Her previous teaching experience included nursing/college students at Penn, pre-med students at Franklin and Marshall, experience in health survey inventories in PA, Department of Health

(1960-61); fellow in medical genetics at Johns Hopkins, and co-author with Victor A. McKusick of a paper on the Ellis-van Creveld (EvC) syndrome (1964), a classic to this day.

Egeland taught required courses for first and second year medical students, plus electives. She worked closely with Dr. Hiram Wiest developing the Family & Community Medicine Department's assignment of each medical student to follow a local family both at home and during medical appointments at TMSHMC. While teaching full-time, Egeland was made project director for a grant awarded to Dean George Harrell. The goal was to address health needs of the local community, and their concerns for the impact of the new teaching hospital (i.e. potential problems between "town and gown" which Dr. Harrell had experienced as a founding Dean elsewhere). Egeland designed the survey interview guides, recruited a team of local women (including the former private nurse for Milton S. Hershey) to conduct home interviews. The analyzed data and recommendations were presented in two monographs, with an opening chapter on the early health care Mr. Hershey provided in Derry Township (See: Egeland, J. A.: *Health Resources Inventory*. 45 pages, 1973, and the *Community Health Survey*, 260 pages, 1974, College of Medicine, The Pennsylvania State University; both in The George T. Harrell Library, TMSHMC). Egeland was the first faculty member to publish a book (a 605 page Amish Mennonite Genealogy, Johns Hopkins Hospital, 1972). She was awarded tenure in 1973.

A new Dean's policy that restricted research to campus prevented planned genetic research among the Amish. Coupled with low salaries after eight years of service resulted in her going on a "leave of absence" and transferring to the Department of Psychiatry, School of Medicine, University of Miami, Miami, FL (1974), There she was offered the unique opportunity of leaving campus as a "scholar-at-large" to conduct full-time research on the genetics of major affective disorders among the Amish (P. I. and project director of the Amish Study, funded 1976). She also had an appointment as Lecturer, then Adjunct Professor of Psychiatry, Department of Psychiatry, School of Medicine, University of Pennsylvania (1976-present) as well as

Adjunct Professor of Psychiatry, University of Massachusetts, School of Medicine, Worchester, MA (1989-2008). Egeland retired in 2006 as a Professor Emerita but returned to active status immediately. She has continued working full-time, insuring that guidelines for patient contact and medical records receive approval (IRB) on an annual basis. Her work became increasingly renowned, international in scope, and received many honors and awards.

Egeland's Amish Study pioneered research discoveries for bipolar affective disorder, a psychiatric condition *not unique to Amish* in prevalence (1.5- 2 % in all populations) or in clinical features and response to treatment. The three most significant breakthroughs have been: (1) The first study world-wide to abandon conventional genetic markers and embrace the new DNA technology to search for a gene for a psychiatric condition (*Nature*, 1987): (2) the first and only investigation to have found a protective gene for bipolar disorder and mapped its location (*PNAS*, 1998); and (3) the first study to discover and map the location of a protective pathway for bipolar affective disorders (*Nature, Molecular Psychiatry*, Nov, 2014). This recent publication was built on her work on Ellis-van Criveld dwarfism in 1964, and represents an initiative to help define the evolution of psychiatric genetics over 50 years.

The Department of Behavioral Science gradually became one of experimental psychology and neuroscience. It later merged with the Department of Anatomy to become first, the Department of Neuroscience and Anatomy, and then the Department of Neural and Behavioral Sciences. Behavioral Science, as an entity, has almost ceased to exist; however, the need (as envisioned by Dr. Harrell) still persists.

DEPARTMENT of BIOLOGICAL CHEMISTRY-- EUGENE DAVIDSON, Ph.D., founding Chair, 1967-88. Dr Davidson was born in 1930. He received his B.S. in chemistry (UCLA) in 1950, and Ph.D. in biochemistry (USC) in 1955. He served (1955-58) as a Research Associate and Instructor in Biological Chemistry at the University of Michigan. He was appointed to Duke University as Assistant Professor in 1958, promoted to Associate Professor in 1962, and to Professor in 1967. He was recruited to TMSHMC in 1967 as Professor and Chair, Department of Biological Chemistry. He concurrently served as Associate Dean for Education, 1975-87.

Davidson was attracted to TMSHMC because of the opportunity to be involved in the establishment of a new medical school; the recruitment of senior faculty and the development of a curriculum. He fully accepted the founding deans' emphasis on teaching as a primary goal. He also recognized the opportunity to develop a strong laboratory research program.

At the first Executive Committee Meeting (composed of department chairs), Dr. Harrell announced that the College of Science had opposed the name Department of Biochemistry in the College of Medicine because they already had a Department of Biochemistry in their College. Dr. Davidson immediately responded by saying "Fine, we will call it the Department of Biological Chemistry." This was viewed as a demonstration of collegial cooperation. They later changed their name to the Department of Biological Chemistry and Molecular Biology. His department was one of the first to develop an outreach program to colleges and universities in Pennsylvania, which was crucial in recruiting graduate students and postdoctoral fellows.

In 1988, Davidson left to be Professor and Chair of Biochemistry and Molecular Biology, Georgetown University Medical Center (GUMC), Washington, DC. He stepped down as Chair at GUMC in 2003, and retired in 2008.

Davidson's vision and goals were quite clear; faculty expertise in the basic areas of biochemistry, i.e. carbohydrate chemistry (Davidson), protein chemistry (Hass), lipid chemistry (Rosenberg), etc. The goal was to ensure excellence, and coverage, in the medical curriculum yet with the goal of research expertise in each of the areas. Davidson was very productive; 200+ scientific publications, 14 book chapters, 2 books, 10 patents, and author of the chapter on carbohydrates in Encyclopedia Britannia.

DEPARTMENT of COMPARATIVE MEDICINE -- C. MAX LANG, D.V.M., DACLAM, founding Chair, 1966-2006.

Dr. Lang was born in Paris, IL on December 29, 1937. He was raised on a farm in east-central IL. He attended local schools, spending the first 6 years in a one room school (1 teacher for 6 grades), then went to a consolidated school system. This school system was relatively small; there were 19 in his high school graduating class.

He attended the University of Illinois, Champaign-Urbana, IL, and transferred to the College of Veterinary Medicine after two years of undergraduate study (the normal was 4+ years), and received his D.V.M. in 1961.

His original career goal was to be a large animal veterinarian. By a twist of fate, this was changed by the military draft (Selective Service System). He entered the US Army Veterinary Corps upon graduation and was assigned to the Walter Reed Army Institute of Research (WRAIR) in Washington, DC as a laboratory animal veterinarian. During this assignment (in addition to his regular duties) he developed, and taught, a course in Laboratory Animal Care for Army technicians, and developed the technology for establishing Specific Pathogen Free animals. He was also asked to start a "VIP" animal clinic which included the pets of President Kennedy, various Cabinet officers, and high ranking military officers.

Upon completion of his military obligation (1961-63), he entered a NIH sponsored postdoctoral fellowship training program in Laboratory Animal Medicine at the Bowman Gray School of Medicine (now the Wake Forest University School of Medicine) in Winston-Salem, NC.

Dr. Lang was recruited to TMSHMC as Assistant Professor and Chair of Comparative Medicine (1966). He was the first faculty appointment recruited by the founding Dean, George T Harrell. He interviewed the week before the Groundbreaking of this new College of Medicine. His first duties were the design and planning for the Animal Resource Facility (composed of the Central Animal Quarters in the Basic Sciences Wing, a separate Animal Research Farm, and existing Gro-Mor Barn. The latter was one of the first 3 farms purchased by Milton Hershey to help support his School.

These design and planning activities extended to the Basic Sciences and Clinical Sciences Wings.

Dr. Lang began to develop his academic and research programs. The Graduate Program in Laboratory Animal Medicine (offering a Master of Science degree to graduate veterinarians) was the first approved by the Graduate School of TPSU for the College of Medicine. During his tenure, there were 57 graduates who went on to achieve specialty certification and serve in academic, military, and pharmaceutical positions with distinction. The program, during his tenure, was supported by NIH Training Grants, the US Army and Air Force, and foreign governments (for their citizen trainees). Four individuals (Lang, Hughes, Landi, and Balk) have been awarded the Charles River Prize in Laboratory Animal Medicine. It is the highest award for a veterinarian in this field, and is awarded annually.

The Animal Resource Facility was designed as a model for humane animal care and research activities. The facilities, veterinary care and husbandry have been cited, in terms of design and management, as a model by both the National Institutes of Health and the National Academy of Sciences. Throughout Lang's tenure the facility was also cited as a model of financial efficiency.

Dr. Lang's research focused on environmental variables that can affect the interpretation of research data and development of animal models for the study of both animal and human diseases. He received over $11 million in peer-reviewed grants (mostly from the NIH) to support his research and training activities. He has 175 peer-reviewed scientific publications, several Visiting Professor invitations, and many invited national and international lectures. He was active in institutional, national and international committees.

In addition to his duties as Chair of Comparative Medicine, he concurrently served as Assistant Dean for Continuing Education, Director of the Cancer Research Center, and administrative responsibility for the George T. Harrell Library. He also assumed responsibility for the "farming" of TMSHMC land. Dr. Lang was active in fund raising and established two University Endowments (each with a book value of more than $1 million) to support developmental research by veterinarians in the Department of Comparative Medicine.

Lang retired in 2006 as the George T. Harrell Professor Emeritus.

DEPARTMENT of HUMANITIES -- A. E. VASTYAN, B.A., B.D., D.Sc. (honorary), founding Chair, 1967-92. He was born June 1, 1928 in Fairport Harbor, OH (died July, 2010). He served in the USAF (1946-47), starting at the age of 18, and rose to the rank of Sergeant. After he left the military, he went to Denison University, OH (on the G. I. bill) where he was elected to Phi Beta Kappa, received Ebenezer Thresher and Julie Barker Sarrett Scholarships for Academic Achievement, and was awarded a B.A. with Honors in 1951. He spent 1951-52 at the University of Southampton, England, with an emphasis on English literature and poetry; worked for a year at the New York Times; returned to Denison University 1953-54 as Instructor in English and Associate Director of Public Information; attended the University of Chicago, (1954-56) to become a minister; and Harvard University/Episcopal Theological School, receiving a B.D. *cum laude.*

His Honors and Awards include the Doctor of Humane Letters in 1979 from the Medical University of South Carolina, and the Alumni Citation in 1986 by Denison University. He participated in many consultantships, seminars and workshops during his academic career.

Mr. Vastyan was an Episcopal Chaplain at the Ohio State University (1957-60). He was also a Chaplain at the University of Texas Medical Branch 1960-67, and concurrently Executive Director of the William Temple Foundation (for Humanistic Studies) 1962-67. During this time he, and a small group of academic chaplains, established the Society for Health and Human Values.

Vastyan was appointed to TMSHMC as Assistant Professor and Acting Chairman of the Department of Humanities (1967-69), promoted to Associate Professor and Chairman (1969-75), and Professor and Chairman (1975-92). He was honored with a University Professorship in Humanities in 1984.

Vastyan established the department with 3 faculty: religion (Vastyan), history (Lurie), and literature/ethics (Clouser). All three were excellent in scholarship and teaching ability. Vastyan developed a course on Dying, Death and Grief, which has been very popular with the medical students. Lurie was a superb and brilliant historian but focused on his area of expertise rather than the broader range of the history of Medicine. He left after a few years. Clouser developed a national reputation in medical ethics and was elected to the Institute of Medicine, National Academy of Science. He had a wry sense of humor; on his tombstone, he has the word "Philosopher", slightly off center and to the left.

Under Vastyan's aegis, the disciplines of ethics, history, literature, philosophy, and religion were incorporated as a required part of the medical curriculum. This was an educational innovation that subsequently spread rapidly throughout medical education in America. Instrumental in the adoption of these disciplines in medical curricula included such organizations as the Society for Health and Human Values, and the Institute of Human Values in Medicine, both of which Vastyan served in leadership positions. Through both organizations, he also served as a consultant on humanistic studies in medicine at some twenty colleges of medicine; and, as a member of the National Board of Consultants of the National Endowment for the Humanities, and at numerous other universities. For six years he served as an advisory board member of the Robert Wood Johnson Clinical Scholars Program.

Vastyan's goals and vision were similar to Dr. Harrell's, i.e., a focus on education and scholarly publications. The department began to wane because of time constraints in the curriculum and the number of courses offered. The requirements were changed to students choosing their own selective courses with a requirement for a minimum number of courses. The department received a boost by the Kienle endowment.

The department established the Center for Humanistic Medicine (CHM) in 1979 to promote ways to restore and enhance care that is both compassionate and technically excellent, emphasizing every patient's individual needs. In 1985, the work of the CHM blossomed when Drs. Kienle, who were both physicians, decided to provide continuing financial support. Following the death of Dr. Jane Kienle in 1991, the CHM was renamed The Doctors Kienle Center for Humanistic Medicine to recognize the contributions of both Drs. Kienles. The Kienles also supported the development of the Doctors Kienle Chair for Humanistic Medicine. The ongoing mission of the Drs. Kienle Center is to support, facilitate, and initiate education and research that will render the delivery of healthcare, both locally and nationally, in a humane fashion. This work has flourished with the support of representatives from many departments throughout the medical center and with that from volunteers in the hospital, medical school, and community.

Vastyan published 28 manuscripts.

DEPARTMENT of MICROBIOLOGY -- FRED RAPP, Ph.D., founding Chair, 1967-90.

Rapp was born in Fulda, Germany March 13, 1929 (died March 20, 2001) and came to the U.S. in 1931 when his family emigrated to get away from the Hitler/Nazi regime. He attended Brooklyn College (B.S., 1951), Albany Medical College (M.S., 1956), and received his Ph.D. from the University of Southern California (USC) in 1958. He remained at USC, first as a Teaching Assistant then as an Instructor, doing research and teaching, then went to Cornell University Medical College (1961-62) as an Assistant Professor. In 1962, he was appointed to the Department of Virology and Epidemiology, Baylor University College of Medicine, Houston, TX as an Associate Professor, later promoted to Professor (1966) and remained there until 1967 when he was appointed Professor and Chairman of the Department of Microbiology, TMSHMC. He also served, concurrently, as Associate Provost and Dean for Health Affairs (1973-80) and Director of the Cancer Research Center (1973-84).

Rapp was a very forceful and energetic individual. He served on many student, college, and university committees. In fact, it is somewhat difficult to summarize his activities because, in his curriculum vitae, he interspersed committee and academic appointments; sometimes duplicating them when he was reappointed or received a renewal grant. He automatically demonstrated an air of authority in both speech and body movements. As a result, in part, he was frequently asked to lecture and serve on numerous national and international committees, which required frequent travel; so much so that the weekly College newsletter was often referred to as "Rapp's Rag."

Rapp's vision and goals were to build a department internationally renowned for research focusing on the role of viruses in cancer, and education (perhaps more so at the graduate and postdoctoral level). He did provide strong oversight of the microbiology portion of the medical student curriculum, ensuring that they learned the core material.

Rapp recruited, primarily, faculty that he had worked with as fellow faculty or post-doctoral fellows at his previous institution (Baylor University College of Medicine). However, not all of them came directly because of a lack of faculty positions or specialized equipment. For example, Drs. Satvir and Judith Tevethia left Baylor for Tufts University because they were a husband wife team (although both were independent investigators) and Rapp had only 1 open position, not 2. When they later came to TMSHMC, they spent their first year preparing lectures and teaching materials for the medical students before re-establishing their highly productive research laboratories. This was indicative of their, and the department's, commitment to teaching.

Rapp had a very productive research career, serving on 50 national and international committees, and a research focus in Herpes viruses, supported largely by the National Cancer Institute, Special Virus Program. He, arguably, developed the best herpesvirus research program in the world with a focus on their oncogenic potential. He published over 360 scientific papers.

RONALD GLASER, Ph.D. (1968, University of Connecticut) was another "delayed" recruitment. When he finished his post-doctoral training (1968-69) at Baylor with a focus on Epstein Barr Virus (EBV), the electron microscopy equipment was not yet installed at Hershey. He spent 1 year at Indiana University (1969-70) then came to Hershey as an Assistant Professor in 1970, promoted to Associate Professor in 1973, and Professor in 1977.

Glaser has a long history of studying the interaction between EBV and epithelial cells as they relate to nasopharyngeal carcinoma (NPC). Because of the extreme difficulty in obtaining stabile EBV genome positive NPC tumor cell lines, he became one of the first to develop an epithelial somatic cell hybrid cell line that was EBV genome–sensitive to study EBV replication in epithelial cells *in vivo*. Since then his research has been devoted to the field of psychoneuroimmunology studying the interactions between the central nervous system, the immune system, and the endocrine system, and how stress modulates the interactions of these systems. His work has focused on stress and herpes-virus latency, vaccine response, wound healing and the role that stress may play as a co-factor in the etiology and progression of malignant disease.

Dr. Glaser is a very productive investigator, publishing more than 300 scientific publications and 26 books and book chapters. He is the recipient of more than $50 million in research grants/contracts.

Dr. Glaser has been recognized for his research by his receipt of a Leukemia and Lymphoma Society Scholar Award and election as a Fellow of the American Association for the Advancement of Science. He served as President of the Psychoneuroimmunology Research Society, and The Academy of Behavioral Medical Research. He was also appointed to serve on the Chronic Fatigue Syndrome Advisory Panel to the Secretary of Health and Human Services.

Dr. Glaser holds the Gilbert and Kathryn Mitchell Endowed Chair in Medicine, and is the Director of the Institute for Behavioral Medicine Research at the Ohio State University Medical Center, Columbus, Ohio.

DEPARTMENT of PHARMACOLOGY -- ELLIOT S(aul) VESELL, M.D.; founding Chair, 1968-2000. He was born in New York City, New York December 24, 1933. His father was a cardiologist, and his uncle a gynecologist, thus exposing him to medicine at an early age. He frequently accompanied his father to medical meetings. His mother encouraged him in the arts by taking him to galleries and museums on weekends. He retained his interest in the arts and literature throughout his professional career.

He graduated with honors from the Phillips Exeter Academy in 1951. He received his A.B. from Harvard College, *magna cum laude,* in 1955 and was elected to Phi Beta Kappa. He received his M.D., *magna cum laude,* in 1959 from Harvard Medical School, where he was a member of the Boyleston Society. He was an Intern, Children's Medical Service, Massachusetts General Hospital (1959-60), Boston, MA; Research Associate and Assistant Physician, Rockefeller University, NY, NY (1960-62),and Assistant Resident Physician, Peter Bent Brigham Hospital, Boston, MA (1962-63). He fulfilled his military obligation as Surgeon, USPHS (Clinical Associate), National Institute of Arthritis and Metabolic Diseases, NIH, Bethesda, MD (1963-65). After completion of his military assignment, he was appointed Head, Section on Pharmacogenetics, Laboratory of Chemical Pharmacology, NIH (1965-68).

In 1968, he was appointed Professor of Medicine, Pharmacology, and Genetics, and Chairman of the Department of Pharmacology, TMSHMC. During this time, he concurrently served as Assistant Dean of Graduate Education (1973-95) and was appointed the Evan Pugh Professor of Pharmacology (1981) and Bernard B. Brodie Professor of Pharmacology (1981). He stepped down as Chair in 2000, but has remained at the institution as an active Emeritus faculty member.

Vesell was a somewhat difficult recruit. He had his own productive research laboratory and secure research funding at the NIH. However, Dr. Harrell persisted because of Vesell's scholarship; research expertise; youthful enthusiasm; capacity for hard work; background discoveries and awards; and vision.

Vesell's goals and vision were instrumental in forming a top tier department, both in research and education. He sought advice from several outstanding departments of pharmacology in the U.S. Using this advice, and his own experiences, he readily achieved his goals and vision. He recruited mainly from former colleagues and others trained at the NIH; he had worked with them and knew their strengths first hand. He purposely selected young investigators from different and diverse areas of pharmacology. Dedication, ingenuity, prior training and tangible evidence of previous research success and productivity were required. The guiding principle for the long-range development of the department arose from his conviction that productive investigators representing diverse scholarly interests could best strengthen and challenge each other. His first faculty appointment was Walter B. Severs, Ph.D., F.C.P. (1968-99). Since Vesell remained at the NIH to complete some research projects, Dr. Severs was somewhat surprised to learn that he was the only faculty member physically on board—and responsible for a good portion of the pharmacology course. Dr. Vesell delivered the first lecture and invited several senior NIH investigators to give others. Dr. Vesell was an excellent mentor, and they persevered, soon being followed by Drs. John Connor and Frank Greene from the NIH. Mentoring of faculty was a strong trait of Dr. Vesell. Throughout Dr. Vesell's tenure, he would take daily walks at noon with his faculty, one at a time, to discuss their teaching and research. Sometimes, the walk was around the medical center or, in case of inclement weather, in the 1,400 foot tunnel connecting the Animal Research Farm with the main building. These settings afforded the opportunity for relaxed, uninterrupted discussions.

Dr. Vesell is well known for his innovative studies on the genetic control of large variations among normal human subjects in metabolism and drug response. They are now credited with constituting the scientific basis for the concept of personalized medicine. These studies were conducted *in vivo* on rates of drug metabolism in normal identical and fraternal twins. He had worked with Dr. Alexander G. Bearn in human biochemical genetics in Dr. Henry Kunkel's laboratory at Rockefeller University on the existence of multiple molecular forms of enzymes. This led to the term "isozyme" and the recognition that these different forms could subserve different functions in the cell. These observations were widely acclaimed and published, after they were initially dismissed as artifactual. Dr. Vesell has authored more than 330 scientific publications, edited several books, and received many national and international awards, including all four major awards in clinical pharmacology in the USA.

Dr. Vesell is an outstanding, internationally recognized scholar respected for his collegiality, cooperation, leadership, and student support.

DEPARTMENT of PHARMACOLOGY -- WALTER B. SEVERS, Ph.D., F.C.P.

Dr. Severs was born in Pittsburgh, PA on June 10,1938. He worked his way through the University of Pittsburgh with the goal of being a pharmacist (B.S. 1960). After graduation, he was working in a pharmacy when a former professor saw him working and expressed surprise that he had not gone on to graduate school. He acted on that advice, and proceeded to get degrees in Pharmacology (M.S. 1963, Ph.D. 1965). During his graduate studies, he was asked to teach pharmacology, on an interim basis, at another university. Although he had considered a career in the pharmaceutical industry, his teaching experience and desire for scientific inquiry led him to a highly competitive position at the NIH as a USPHS Postdoctoral Fellow in the Laboratory of Chemical Pharmacology, NHLBI (sponsor: Dr Bernard B. Brodie).

Dr. Severs' research interests focused on angiotensin and vasopressin pharmacology; hypertension; antihypertensive drugs; neural regulation of the cardiovascular system; neuroendocrinology of salt/water balance; circumventricular organs; central actions of aldosterone; and histamine metabolism and function. His research was well-funded by the NIH and NASA. He published more than 220 peer-reviewed scientific manuscripts. He received many national and international honors and awards for his research.

He was a superb educator at all levels; local, medical students, graduate students, postdoctoral fellows and the world-wide web. Dr. Severs also served on many college and university committees. Dr. Severs was a superb, productive scholar and friend to many. He retired in 1999.

DEPARTMENT of PHYSIOLOGY-- HOWARD E. MORGAN, M.D., founding Chair, 1967-87. He was born October 8, 1927 in Bloomington, IL (died March 2, 2009). He attended Illinois Wesleyan University in Bloomington for one year (1944-45) before transferring to the Johns Hopkins University, receiving his M.D. in 1949. His original intention was to become an obstetrician-gynecologist, a career he began on the house staff of the hospital of Vanderbilt University (1949-53). The following year (1953-54) he was an Instructor in these disciplines. He then became a Fellow for a year in medical research in the unit of the Howard Hughes Institute in the Department of Physiology at Vanderbilt (1954-55). But, the following year he was back in obstetrics-gynecology as Assistant Chief on that service on active duty in the US Army Station at Ft Campbell, KY (1955-57). He then returned to Vanderbilt, and for the next ten years (1957-67) he was an investigator in the Hughes Institute, with faculty rank that progressed from Assistant Professor (1959—62), to Associate Professor (1962-66), and Professor (1966-67). He took a leave of absence (June/1960-September/1961) to further his research capabilities at the Department of Biochemistry, Cambridge University, Cambridge England. He was further honored by appointment as a scholar of the Howard Hughes Medical Institute.

In 1967, Dr. Morgan became the first Professor and Chairman of the Department of Physiology in the new College of Medicine, The Pennsylvania State University, Hershey, PA. It was very clear during his recruitment that his goal was to establish a high quality, productive research department that had a strong commitment to teaching. He was becoming active in the review of NIH grant applications and, using that information, recruited individuals with a high potential for research, but also in the various areas of his discipline. A somewhat reserved, but pragmatic individual, one of his favorite quotes was "every tub has to sit on its own bottom." He encouraged his young, developing faculty to work in laboratories abroad that were on the "cutting edge" of technology.

Dr. Morgan was awarded the Evan Pugh Professor of Physiology (1974-87) and the J. Lloyd Huck Professor of Physiology (1986-87). He also served as the Associate Dean for Research, TMSHMC

(1973-87). He was very good in that role but it was obviously a stretch of his time, given his other activities. When asked why he served in that role since it was a lot of work and took too much time, his response was he did not want anyone else to do it!

He was strongly committed to the education of medical and graduate students and postdoctoral students. He was very talented in being able to make them think about what they were learning and how to apply that information. He was also quite pragmatic in his approach to the learning material. As we approached the beginning of the first class, we were struggling with the assignment of class hours for each required course; the number of hours requested by the various departments were clearly in excess of the hours available and no one was willing to budge. Finally, the Dean – in exasperation – said I am going to ask you one more time the minimum number of hours required to teach your subject and I will start with Physiology. Morgan, who was obviously becoming bored with the whole matter, said "I can teach it in about 45 minutes; I don't know how much they will learn, but I can teach it in about 45 minutes." That broke the deadlock, and we returned to a more reasonable discussion.

Dr. Morgan was internationally regarded as one of the greatest experimental cardiologists of this century. His research focused on the physiological regulation of intermediary metabolism. His early studies investigated the metabolism of glucose and glycogen. In association with Dr James Robert (Bob) Neely, they developed the isolated perfused working heart preparation from adult rats for these metabolic studies. Later in his research career, Morgan's interest shifted to identification of factors that control growth of the heart and that can lead to cardiac hypertrophy. His strong commitment to excellence in heart research, his clear vision for blending the basic sciences with clinical cardiology, and his deep devotion to helping young cardiovascular scientists reach their potential demonstrated his outstanding ability in the creative organization of medical research.

He wrote more than 250 scientific articles. His work was named three times as a "Citation Classic," a paper with more than 500 citations in published research for each article.

Another important feature of Dr. Morgan's career was his association with scientific journals. Beginning with the Editorial Board of the *American Journal of Physiology* (1967-73), he became editor of *Physiological Reviews* (1973-78), associate editor of the *American Journal of Physiology: Endocrinology and Metabolism* (1979-81), and editor of the *American Journal of Physiology: Cell Physiology* (1981-84). For much of this time he served on the American Physiological Society Publications Committee (1979-85; chairman, 1981-85). Other journals for which he provided editorial assistance include *Circulation Research, Journal of Biological Chemistry, Journal of Cardiovascular Pharmacology and Journal of Molecular and Cellular Cardiology*. These editorial endeavors obviously enhanced his knowledge of the discipline and, in turn, enabled him to be on the cutting edge of research innovation and education stimulation.

Dr. Morgan served as President of the American Physiological Society, President of the American Heart Association, President of the International Society for Heart Research, and the founding President of the International Academy of Cardiovascular Sciences. He served as coordinator of the US/USSR exchange program dealing with cardiovascular biology and medicine for 20 years. He was a member of the Institute of Medicine/National Academy of Sciences, and the recipient of the Abigail A Geisinger Award; the Award of Merit, Distinguished Achievement Award and Gold Heart Award from the American Heart Association; Carl J. Wiggers Award and Ray G. Daggs Award from the American Physiological Society; and the Peter Harris Award for outstanding contributions to Cardiovascular Research by the International Society for Heart Research. Dr. Morgan was a consultant to the Reynolds Foundation, Whitaker Foundation, and the Bugher Foundation. This global recognition demonstrates the widespread admiration and affection in which he was held throughout the world.

Dr. Morgan retired from The Pennsylvania State University in 1987 to become the Senior Vice President for Research, Director of Research, Sigfried and Janet Weis Center for Research, Geisinger Clinic, Danville, PA.

DEPARTMENT of PHYSIOLOGY -- LEONARD S. (Jim) JEFFERSON, Ph.D.

Dr. Jefferson is one of the founding faculty members of the Department of Physiology. He was born January 14, 1939 in Maysvile, KY.

His father was a farmer and had limited formal education. He had hoped that his son would remain on the farm. He credits his parents with developing a very strong work ethic. His mother graduated from high school and strongly encouraged her sons to further their education. He finally convinced his father that if he went to the nearby Eastern Kentucky University, he could continue helping with the farm during the school year and in the summers. In college, he majored in Chemistry/Biology and received the B.S. in 1961. He had a strong interest in the sciences, and had excelled in chemistry so he decided to enroll at Vanderbilt University. He was interviewed as a prospective medical student by Dr. Rollo Park (an M.D. and chair of Physiology). Park convinced him to enroll in the M.D./Ph.D program. His father accepted that since he was going to be a "doctor". He completed the first two years of medical school, and then worked full time on his Ph.D. studies. He knew then, that he was far more interested in research than the practice of medicine. Upon receiving the Ph.D. in 1966, he decided to continue his research rather than complete the requirements for the M.D. degree. It was a decision that he never regretted.

His research was on Cyclic AMP with a focus on mediating the actions of insulin to suppress glucose production by the liver. The department at Vanderbilt, at the time, was just beginning to attain the level of prominence it enjoys today. In addition to Rollo Park and his wife Janie, other faculty included Howard Morgan, Earl Sutherland, David Regen, John Exton and others. Sutherland had recently received the Nobel Prize for his discovery of cyclic AMP. When Jefferson finished his Ph.D. (1966), Dr. Park was very keen on sending promising postdoctoral fellows to other countries. Jefferson applied for, and received a USPHS Fellowship to study in the Department of Biochemistry, Cambridge, England under Dr. Asher Korner. He had planned to stay two years, but Korner accepted the chair of Biochemistry at Sussex, and Dr. Jefferson did not want to be involved in a move. Dr. Morgan had accepted the chair of Physiology at Hershey and offered Jefferson a position. Since the labs had not yet been built, Morgan arranged for Jefferson to complete his postdoc at Vanderbilt.

Dr. Jefferson was appointed to the faculty in 1967 as an Instructor, promoted to Assistant Professor (1968-72); promoted to Associate Professor (1972-75); and Professor in 1975. He was appointed Chair of the Department of Cellular and Molecular Physiology in 1988. He concurrently served as the Associate/Vice Dean for Research (1990-2001). He was awarded the Evan Pugh Professorship in 1996.

Dr. Jefferson has had a productive research career and received several honors and awards, including awards from the American Diabetes Association and the Juvenile Diabetes Foundation.

DEPARTMENT of PHYSIOLOGY – ANTHONY E. PEGG, Ph.D.

Dr. Anthony E. Pegg is one of the founding faculty members of the Department of Physiology (1975-2012). He was born April 13, 1942 in Matlock, Derbyshire, England, and became a U.S. citizen in 1983.

Dr. Pegg was educated in the English system, and attended the University of Cambridge, England on a scholarship. He received his B.A. (Natural Sciences) in 1963; M.A. (Natural Sciences) in 1964; and Ph.D. (Biochemistry) in 1966. Dr. Pegg was a Postdoctoral Fellow in the Department of Pharmacology, Johns Hopkins University Medical School (1966-68), working with Dr. Guy Williams-Ashman, who had recently transferred from the University of Chicago to Hopkins. Williams-Ashman was an expert on the reproductive tract and how it was affected by hormones. Pegg elected to study polyamines in the prostate where their synthesis is hormonally regulated. But no one knew much about the biosynthesis of polyamines in mammalian tissues. They were the first to discover two key enzymes in the biosynthetic pathway which were decarboxylases. At this point he considered himself to be a biochemist but also, to some extent, a physiologist. His primary research interests were: how polyamines mediated signals from hormones which was physiologically oriented, and DNA repair and its importance in mutating cells from environmental insults.

Dr. Pegg had visited Hershey during his fellowship training at Hopkins and Dr. Morgan (founding Chair of Physiology) approached him about joining his faculty. However, he felt an obligation to return to England since they had paid for his education. He returned to England to teach and do research at the University of London (1969-74). He was recruited to Hershey as an Associate Professor of Physiology in 1975.

Dr. Pegg's goal was to run his own research laboratory studying carcinogens and cancer, with a focus on polyamines and DNA repair. His research was well funded by highly competitive research grants. He published over 600 peer reviewed scientific papers and gave many national and international lectures. Dr. Pegg received many honors and awards for his scholarship; most notably the endowed Evan Pugh and J. Lloyd Huck Professorships and the Henry Hood Research Award for Outstanding Achievement in Biomedical Research.

Dr. Pegg is a gifted scientist with a scholarly insight. He was never one to be bothered with administrative trivia, but a willing collaborator and participant.

CHAPTER 6

CLINICAL SCIENCE DEPARTMENTS

DEPARTMENT of ANESTHESIOLOGY -- ALLEN E. YEAKEL, M.D. was the founding Chair (1970-76), He was born March 21, 1921 in Fair Oaks, PA. He fulfilled his military obligation in the U.S. Navy Reserve as a Lt, j.g., Radar Maintenance Officer (1944-46). He then returned to Carnegie Institute, Pittsburgh (1946-47) before applying to medical school. He received his M.D. from the University of Pennsylvania in 1951. Dr. Yeakel completed an internship (1951-52) at the Philadelphia General Hospital, Philadelphia, PA; and a residency in general practice (1952-53) at Sacred Heart Hospital, Norristown, PA.

After his residency, he entered the general practice of medicine (1953-59) in Bechtelsville, PA with hospital appointments at Pottstown Hospital and Memorial Hospital, both in Pottstown, PA. He returned (1959) to the Hospital of the University of Pennsylvania for a residency in anesthesiology. Dr.Yeakel began his academic career as Assistant Instructor in Anesthesiology, University of Pennsylvania School of Medicine. He then went to the West Virginia University Medical Center, Division of Anesthesiology, as an Instructor in 1961. He was quickly promoted to Assistant Professor later in 1961, then to Associate Professor in 1965, and to Professor in 1969.

Dr. Yeakel was recruited to TMSHMC by Dr. John Waldhausen, Professor and Chair, Department of Surgery. It was originally thought that Anesthesiology would be a Division of Surgery (as it was at West Virginia) but the decision was made to make it a separate department. Dr. Yeakel was excited about the teaching and patient care opportunities but somewhat hesitant about the emphasis on research. In his previous academic career, he had produced 9 publications, all of which were descriptive reports; he had not received any external funding. He was surprised that he was even considered for the position, given his lack of research credentials.

Dr. Yeakel was a modest, introspective individual and approached his new position with some hesitation. He promised his wife that he would return to private practice if he became dissatisfied with the growth of the department within 5 years. He even bought a home half way between Lancaster and Hershey so that he could change positions without having to move his home.

His attempts to build a department of his dreams were often met with frustration. A favorite quote of his was by Dr. Joseph Priestley, a renowned anesthesiologist: "*I have a tolerably good habit of circumspection with regards to facts, but as to conclusions from them, I am not apt to be very confident.*" This may have been indicative of his own self- assessment.

Dr. Yeakel approached his appointment with vigor and enthusiasm; recruiting staff and faculty; buying and testing equipment; designing the anesthesia record; developing the curricula for second and third year medical students; planning the residency program, including applications for approval by the AAMC; etc.

He was a stickler for detail. This trait avoided at least one potential disaster. About a week before the hospital opened, he sensed that something was wrong with the oxygen lines. He took samples of the gas to the Department of Biological Chemistry and found that the gas sample was helium, not oxygen, that had been used to test for leaks, and the contractor had failed to flush the helium out of the lines. They opened all of the lines in the medical center to flush the lines and it was the next day before they were getting 100% oxygen. They had the same problem with nitrous oxide and flushed those lines as well.

They only had 4 staff anesthesiologists by the second year, and 7 in the third year. The faculty were very active, lecturing during the pharmacology course and introducing third year students to clinical anesthesia for 2 weeks during their surgical rotation, participating in Continuing Education programs, etc. They were clearly at, or beyond, their limit. There was some pressure to hire nurse anesthetists, but Yeakel refused because that was a condition of his appointment; he firmly believed that the type of anesthesia required in a referral/teaching hospital required physician anesthesiologists. They were asked to provide on-call rotations in the Emergency Room. Again, he refused because they were not trained in that specialty and he did not have the manpower.

Dr. Yeakel developed a system to ensure efficient and adequate anesthesia support for all surgical procedures, including average, minimum, and maximum times to complete the surgical procedure. Surgeons were also required to file a 3 x 5 card for every planned elective case. Anesthesiology then added the estimated time, met with the O.R. Coordinator and, using a data base, generated the next day's operating schedule. Although a good idea, others involved resisted what they saw as a lack of flexibility.

Another frustration was recruitment of faculty. Dr. Yeakel wanted to establish a Division to maintain the integrity and safety of all equipment, and had an outstanding candidate for the position. But, the Business Manager of the medical center said "No, I don't have the money." This was repeated when he tried to establish a formal pain control service and multidisciplinary pain clinic. He probably should have made his requests to the Dean rather than the Business Manager.

Research was slow to develop, but he was able to recruit Dr Michael Nahrwold (brother of Dr David Nahrwold in the Department of Surgery) from the NIH to establish a laboratory to study the effects of anesthetic agents on neurotransmitters. Yeakel believed that he missed some opportunities to develop a strong research program. His former Chief at Penn called Yeakel a few times with suggestions of research oriented anesthesiologists, but later Yeakel realized he was so involved that he did not take advantage of these opportunities.

In retrospect, Dr. Yeakel believed that he had unwittingly antagonized people who could impede the progress of the Department. For whatever the reason, he was doing what he sincerely believed was right and in a manner that would yield results. He resigned in 1976 to do what he enjoyed best—taking care of patients full time. He then joined a private anesthesia practice, Lancaster General Hospital, Lancaster, PA.

DEPARTMENT of ANESTHESIA – JULIEN F. BIEBUYCK, M.B., Ch.B., D.Phil.

Dr. Biebuyck was born Feb 2, 1935 in Pietermaritzburg, Natal, South Africa, and attended Durban Preparatory School for Boys, Durban High School, and Maritzburg College (1944-52), all in Natal, South Africa. He attended medical school at the University of Cape Town. Following his internship and residency, he practiced for two years as a General Practitioner, concentrating on Obstetrics, Pediatrics, and Anesthesia in his hometown of Pietermaritzburg. He then returned to the University of Cape Town and the Groote Schuur Hospital in 1966 to complete a formal residency in Anesthesiology.

During his clinical residency he initiated a basic research program (in collaboration with the Liver Research Group: Hepatologists and Liver Transplant Surgeons) to address a world-wide increase in liver failure following surgery. Most of these patients had received the anesthetic agent halothane. His research was to determine the causes and mechanisms of liver damage following anesthesia using halothane. This research led to his selection as a Nuffield Research Fellow to study at Trinity College in Oxford University, England. His research at Oxford was conducted in the Metabolic Research Laboratory of the Radcliffe Infirmary under the direction of Sir Hans Krebs who had received the Nobel Prize for Physiology and Medicine in 1952.

Following the award of the D.Phil. degree for his research at Oxford, Dr. Biebuyck was recruited to Harvard Medical School as a Medical Foundation Fellow and as an Assistant Professor in the Department of Anesthesiology, Massachusetts General Hospital

(MGH). In addition to his focus on Neuroanesthesiology, he established the Anesthesia Metabolic Research Laboratory in the Department of Anesthesia at MGH and the affiliated Shriners Burns Institute. His research involved the alterations in hepatic synthetic functions, such as gluconeogenesis following burn injury, and the changes in brain neurotransmitters during anesthesia and hypoxia.

In 1977, Dr. Biebuyck was recruited to the College of Medicine, The Pennsylvania State University as Chair of the Department of Anesthesiology, a position he held for twenty years, until 1997. He developed a nationally competitive department, with seven Divisions. He established several major laboratories funded by the National Institutes of Health (NIH) to study: the mechanisms of Sleep and Coma; the Artificial Lung; Cardiac Function during anesthesia; and Malignant Hypothermia. By 1990, his department ranked in the top ten of anesthesiology departments nationally in NIH funding. Dr Biebuyck established the first Cognitive Science and Simulation Development Laboratory in the nation in collaboration with the Applied Research Laboratory of Penn State at University Park, PA. He also established the first Palliative Care Program in a Department of Anesthesia, and one of the early palliative care programs in the nation. Within operating room anesthesiology, the sections of cardiac anesthesiology, pediatric anesthesiology, and regional anesthesia gained national prominence and recognition.

In the discipline of Anesthesiology, Dr. Biebuyck held several positions of national leadership: Editor of the Journal of Anesthesiology, President of the Society of Academic Anesthesiology Chairs (125 Department Chairs in the United States), Chair of the Committee for Research of the American Society of Anesthesiologists, a member of the Board of Directors of the Foundation for Anesthesia Research in Rochester, MN, and Associate Examiner for the American Board of Anesthesiology. He also served six years as Chair of the Clinical Sciences Publications Committee of the American Physiological Society.

Dr. Biebuyck was very active in leadership roles at TMSHMC and the University at large. He was a member of the search committee for the University President, served on the University

Future Committee, and chaired the search committee for the Dean and CEO of the College of Medicine and TMSHMC. He chaired the search committees for several department chairs at the medical center. He was awarded the Eric A. Walker named and endowed Chair in 1985.

In recognition of his interest and expertise in academic matters, Dr. Biebuyck was appointed Associate Dean for Academic Affairs in 1991, and Senior Associate Dean for Academic Affairs in 1996. He was active in national activities of the Association of American Medical Colleges (AAMC) for more than fifteen years. In 2001, he was appointed as a Robert G. Petersdorf Scholar-in-Residence at the AAMC in Washington, D.C., and remained active as a senior consultant for several years. In 2012, Dr Biebuyck spearheaded the formation of the Penn State College of Medicine Emeritus Faculty Organization, and served as its first President in 2013-14.

DEPARTMENT of FAMILY AND COMMUNITY MEDICINE -- THOMAS L LEAMAN, M.D.; founding Chair, 1967-87. He was born August 18, 1923 in Lancaster, PA and reared in nearby Lititz. He had, and to some extent still has, the basic characteristics of the Pennsylvania Dutch which include frugality, cleanliness, and an unquenchable work ethic. His father was a grocer. His father had been a cigar maker but developed a grocery store so his son would have a good occupation.

Dr. Leaman graduated from Lititz High School in 1941, and entered Gettysburg College. During his second year, he was "called up" by the U.S. Army and began basic training. There was a national shortage of health care professionals, and he was one of a group of soldiers chosen, by an aptitude examination, to attend an intensive pre-medical program at Baylor University in Waco, TX. This training consisted of three weeks of concentrated instruction, then one week off, and then the cycle continued. The imminence of war had brought about the development of new institutions to meet this growing crises. Resources were stretched. His wife, for example, was pregnant and he was pleased that her obstetrician was none other than the

Chair of Obstetrics himself. It was only later that he realized that the chair was actually the entire Department of Obstetrics—there were no others—the school was just being organized! The program at Baylor was then followed by a condensed medical school course at Southwestern Medical School in Dallas, TX.

When the war ended, Leaman transferred to the George Washington University School of Medicine in Washington, D.C. After receiving his medical degree (1948), he went to the Lancaster General Hospital, Lancaster, PA for a one-year rotating internship. Upon completion in 1949, he sought a small town in urgent need of a general practice physician and chose Hershey, a town of about 2,500 people.

Several years later, he was recalled by the Army, this time as a physician and an officer. He was sent to the Air University at Randolph Field, San Antonio, TX. After two years, he returned to Hershey and continued his solo practice. He began looking for courses that he might take to enhance his knowledge of family medicine. He took several courses in Philadelphia, but they were not really helpful. He was restless and thought perhaps he should go overseas to a third world country. He consulted with his Episcopal Bishop who assured him that if God wanted him to be elsewhere, "He" would let him know.

On August 23, 1963 The Pennsylvania State University announced plans to establish a medical school in Hershey.

The biggest problem in Hershey was that the physicians were overrun with patients. The Pennsylvania Academy of Family Physicians asked Drs. Edward Kowalewski and Leaman to tell this new Dean about their problem. They did so and the new Dean responded that he intended to start the first program in the country of Family and Community Medicine and, if they were interested, they could apply to him. There were three conditions: bring their practice into the medical center; accept an academic salary; and get one year of experience working with medical students and residents. Leaman applied, but to meet the requirements, he needed a partner.

Hiram Weist, a family practitioner from East Petersburg, PA met all of the criteria. They formed a legal partnership. They visited every medical school they could find that had expressed any interest in family medicine; in the USA, Canada, Great Britain, and the Netherlands.

Leaman had read the basic text *The Doctor, the Patient, and His Illness* by Michael Balint who was teaching in England, and wanted to meet him. He was permitted to do so, and attended several of his sessions. He found those to be very helpful.

When the medical center opened in the Fall of 1967, the Department of Family and Community Medicine was ready. They had determined that Family and Community Medicine should begin in the first year of medical school in order to provide students four years to be involved with a family.

The Department realized they had done nothing to ease the shortage of physicians in the area. They then found two registered nurses who were interested in learning to become family practice assistants. The Department provided them with both practical clinical experience and the necessary medical courses. This was so successful that they developed an accredited Physician Assistant program, graduating 350 students during the next decade.

Family and Community Medicine was growing rapidly. It was recognized as a specialty of medicine. Leaman was active in the leadership of this new specialty. Hershey was the first academic department of Family and Community Medicine in the country. Leaman helped to found the Society of the Teachers of Family and Community Medicine, and was elected President. He also helped to form the Association of Chairs of Family Medicine, and remained active in this specialty until his retirement in 1991.

In retrospect, Leaman marvels at all that was accomplished through bold imagination, new teaching methods, and establishing novel programs involving hundreds of people.

Various site visitors and other professionals often suggested that Dr. Harrell was building a medical school for general practitioners, rather than a modern, progressive medical school. This misperception was further enhanced by an article (not condoned by Dr. Harrell) describing the new medical center and titled "Handbags and Hearts". Dr. Harrell strongly argued against this analogy. He insisted that

Family & Community Medicine would have the same rigor and expertise as other clinical specialties and he predicted that our graduates would pursue specialties in the same percentage as other top medical schools, but those choosing Family and Community Medicine would be better trained; although he admitted that the article generated a lot of publicity.

DEPARTMENT of MEDICINE -- GRAHAM H. JEFFRIES, M.B., Ch.B., D.Phil., MACP was the founding Chair (1969-88). He was born in Barmera, South Australia on May 31, 1929. His father was a farmer and because of a severe drought, the family moved to New Zealand when he was eight years of age. He proved to be an outstanding student who aspired to be a physician from the age of 12. He completed his medical degree (B.Med.Sc.,1949) and postgraduate (M.B.,Ch.B,.1953) in New Zealand with academic distinction. Although he received his degree in 1953, he actually completed all of the requirements six months previously. He was chosen to be a Rhodes Scholar and, at Oxford University, England completed his D. Phil. (1955) In the laboratory of Sir Howard Florey who had received the Nobel Prize for his research which resulted in the first production of penicillin for clinical use. He was a House Physician, Oxford Hospitals (Sir George Pickering) 1955-57, and House Physician, Royal Postgraduate Medical School, Hammersmith Hospital 1957-58.

While in England, he met Elizabeth Jones, an American who was also studying in the U.K. They were married in 1955. In 1958, Dr. Jeffries accepted a position in the Gastroenterology Program at New York Hospital-Cornell Medical Center (NYH/Cornell). He was a very productive, outstanding clinical investigator whose work was published in prestigious journals. He was elected to membership in prestigious medical and scientific societies in recognition of his work. In 1968, he was appointed as Chief of Gastroenterology at NYH/Cornell. In addition to his scientific expertise, he also demonstrated a sincere commitment to the education of medical students, postgraduate residents, and trainees. This is a commitment that he has maintained throughout his medical career.

In November, 1968, Dr. Jeffries was contacted by Dr. George T. Harrell (founding Dean of TPSU College of Medicine), and asked if he would be interested in being considered for the position of Chair of Medicine. Dr. Jeffries had always had a long-term goal of being a Chair of Medicine, but thought the opportunity would not arise for another 10 years or so. At the time of Dr. Harrell's inquiry, Jeffries knew little about the new medical center being planned and very little about Hershey or the Central Pennsylvania area. As the recruitment proceeded, he became increasingly interested, but had many questions about how the program would be developed, where the patients would come from, how difficult it might be to recruit faculty to a semi-rural area, etc. A senior colleague at Cornell advised him "If you see this as an opportunity that will be a life-long challenge, you must accept; if you view this as a stepping stone to another position, then you must remain at Cornell." Dr. Jeffries gave the matter considerable thought. He knew that he would not have time to pursue his research interests that he had developed into a well-staffed and well-funded program at Cornell. However, he also knew that he would be able to start a brand new department and to teach and mentor hundreds, if not thousands, of medical students and postgraduate trainees over the course of a life time commitment to the growth and development of the College of Medicine, TMSHMC, TPSU.

He accepted Dr. Harrell's offer and arrived in Hershey in July, 1969 as the first academic clinical faculty member. The pioneer class of medical students was about to begin their third academic year and start their clinical rotations. Dr. Jeffries was concerned about where they would receive this clinical training since the Teaching Hospital would not open for another year. Under Dr. Jeffries' leadership, the staff of Harrisburg Hospital warmly received the students, and did a superb job of providing them with excellent clinical experiences in the various specialties.

In addition to his teaching, there was also the need to build a department. Recruiting of faculty was a high priority, and he had to balance this priority with his very heavy teaching responsibilities.

Dr. Jeffries served as Chair of the Department of Medicine for 20 years. Over that time, he built a strong department in teaching, patient care, and research. When he stepped down as Chair, the department was performing well in all of these areas. In addition to his administrative duties, he kept, and met, his commitment to the education and training of medical students, residents, and fellows. Dr. Jeffries is a gifted, and articulate, lecturer in both small groups and one-on-one teaching, he has never failed to inspire and motivate his students. These talents have persisted throughout his career, and continue to the present.

After he relinquished the chairmanship, Dr. Jeffries became an active member of the Division of Gastroenterology and performed, with grace, as a member of the team but no longer boss. He became much more active in patient care and has continued his passion for teaching. Also, he has actively taught in the first and second year curricula as needed.

Dr. Jeffries' commitment to students has been recognized by the creation of special programs in his honor. Among these is the Graham and Elizabeth Jeffries Scholarship, which provides partial financial assistance to a select group of students each year. Another is the Graham and Elizabeth Jeffries International Health Fund which supports elective medical experiences in developing countries. One of Dr. Jeffries most enjoyable activities is interviewing prospective medical students. As he has reduced his time spent in clinical activities in recent years, he has had even more time to devote to these efforts. He keeps track of all the people he interviews, and follows up to see if they came to Hershey for medical school.

In part, or because of his dedication to teaching and patient care, some have criticized him for not devoting more of his time to faculty recruitment. Others have criticized his lack of attention to the administrative side of his duties as a Chair of a major clinical department. On the other hand, there can be no doubt of his lasting legacy as a devoted and highly effective teacher and mentor for close to two generations of medical students, residents, and trainees.

DEPARTMENT of MEDICINE, DIVISION of CARDIOLOGY-- JAMES GAULT, M.D., founding Chief (1970-74)

Gault spent his formative years in rural Tennessee. That obviously was a factor when he was being recruited to Hershey. He graduated from Amherst College in 1957, with a major in Biology and a minor in English, but he wrote his thesis in biochemistry. The choice of a career in medicine was largely due to his strong interest in science and humanitarian beliefs. He chose Cornell for medical school, receiving the M.D. degree in 1961. After graduation he began an Internal Medicine residency and developed a special interest in Cardiology although he admits that cardiology, at that time, consisted mainly of listening to the heart with a stethoscope and reading an electrocardiogram. He knew that he wanted more training in cardiology, and was accepted by the NIH. This was a period of "powerhouse" research in cardiology. Dr Eugene Braunwald was there at the time and he is considered by many to be one of the fathers of modern cardiology. It was a very productive research program, probably one of the most productive in the country. When Braunwald went to San Diego, Gault was one of 10 to go with him.

Dr. Gault was invited to look at Hershey as the first Chief of the Division of Cardiology. He saw that as an intellectual challenge and the opportunity to build a program from the ground up. Cardiology was rapidly evolving as a specialty, and the proposed space was not prepared for changing technology, interventional procedures, or intensive patient care. However, he was able to improvise and develop a quality program. He had excellent recruiting skills, and many of his faculty went on to leadership positions.

Perhaps his greatest struggle was trying to develop a futuristic program in a facility that was dated when it was built. It was also a time of dwindling funding for cardiology research and training programs.

He left to develop a private cardiology practice in Lancaster which became one of the largest 10 in the U.S. His student, resident, and young investigator experiences have given him an unique insight into the changing role of medicine.

DEPARTMENT of MEDICINE, DIVISION of CARDIOLOGY -- DAVID M. LEAMAN, M.D.

Dr. Leaman was born April 24, 1935 in Lancaster, PA. He was uncertain about his career goals when he graduated from high school. He worked as a laborer for three years before deciding to go to college. He started at Franklin and Marshall, but found it to be a very unfriendly place, especially the faculty attitudes towards students. He transferred to Eastern Mennonite College to complete his pre-med requirements, and received his B.A. degree in 1960. He chose Temple for his medical education, receiving the M.D. degree in 1964.

His original plans were to be a family doctor. However, he began to question the vast quantity of knowledge required for family medicine. He decided to do a rotating internship. He did his internship (1964-65) and residency (1965-66) at the Mary Hitchcock Hospital, Hanover, NH. His residency was interrupted by military service. He served in the Public Health Service in Alaska (1966-68). He completed his residency (1968-69) at the Medical Center Hospital of Vermont, Burlington, VT. He was inspired to go there because a former advisor at Hitchcock had been appointed as Chief of Medicine. He then completed a Fellowship in Cardiopulmonary Diseases (1969-71) at the Hospital of Vermont.

Dr. Leaman was appointed Assistant Professor of Medicine, Division of Cardiology, TMSHMC in 1971. He was promoted to Associate Professor in 1977, and to Professor in 1984, He had several leadership positions in the Division of Cardiology, including: Director, Heart Station (1971-73); Director, Cardiac Catheterization Laboratory (1973-85); Director, Clinical Cardiology (1982-85); and Acting, and Chief, Division of Cardiology (1984-95). He is highly respected for his expertise in clinical cardiology.

He has received many honors and awards for his contributions to his field of expertise at both the local and state levels. He was the first recipient of the endowed American Heart Association, South Central Pennsylvania Chapter Professor of Medicine.

DEPARTMENT of MEDICINE, DIVISION of CARDIOLOGY – ROBERT ZELIS, M.D.

Dr. Zelis was born August 5, 1939 in Perth Amboy, NJ and grew up in Chicopee Falls, MA. He graduated *cum laude* from the University of Massachusetts (Chemistry) and received his M.D. degree with Honors from the University of Chicago. He completed his internship and one year of residency at Beth Israel Hospital in Boston, MA. He then entered the USPHS as a Clinical Associate in Cardiology at the NIH, under the leadership of Dr. Eugene Braunwald who is considered to be one of the fathers of modern cardiology.

Dr. Zelis developed an interest in science while in junior high school. He was initially interested in becoming an engineer. As a senior in high school, he decided that he wanted to pursue a career in medical research. His first two publications resulted from research he did while in medical school. He did not do research during his residency. His two years at the NIH in Dr. Braunwald's program were very productive, and he continued to be productive throughout his career. He has been an author or co-author of over 350 publications. He has been a member of many prestigious national medical and scientific organizations including a term as President of the American Federation for Clinical Research, and a term as Vice President of the American Society for Clinical Investigation.

Dr. Zelis began his academic career in 1968 at the University of California, Davis School of Medicine as an Assistant Professor of Medicine and Physiology. The medical school accepted its first class that year and he was very active in teaching cardiovascular sciences in the fully integrated preclinical and clinical curriculum at the new medical school. Another major priority for the new medical school was to attract referral patients to the Medical School Teaching Hospital. The major teaching hospital was named the Sacramento Medical Center. It had previously been named the Sacramento County Hospital and, under that name, had not been a referral center. The efforts to attract patients involved clinical faculty going out and giving talks and updates in their field to a wide geographic area in an effort to build up referral patterns. He was promoted to Associate Professor in 1972 and held several leadership positions.

In 1974, Zelis was contacted by Dr. Graham Jeffries (Chair of Medicine) regarding the Chief of Cardiology position. At first, he didn't think he would be interested. But then he was visited by Dr. Wayne Bardin, founding Chief of Endocrinology, who convinced Zelis to visit Hershey to take a look. Dr. Zelis' visit went very well and he was impressed with the faculty, space, and facilities, especially the new purpose built Medical Center Hospital. Dr. Zelis accepted the position and arrived in Hershey in the summer of 1974 with an appointment as Professor of Medicine and Physiology. He was given a mandate by the Dean to develop a nationally recognized academic Cardiology program to complement those of Howard Morgan in cardiovascular physiology and John Waldhausen in cardiac surgery. As he pursued his own research on circulatory control mechanisms in heart failure, he recruited and mentored a number of trainees and young faculty who have expanded the field. He was recognized for these efforts when he was awarded the Howard Palmer Mentoring Award by The Pennsylvania State University in 1997. He was also honored by the University of Chicago Division of Medical and Biological Sciences with the Distinguished Achievement Award in 2004.

In addition to his impressive research accomplishments, he has been very active in a variety of faculty leadership positions, especially in the medical school curriculum. In 1988, he assumed direction of the Principles of Internal Medicine course, and was a leader in integrating it with other second year courses. In 1996, he was a member of the small task force that reformulated the preclinical curriculum that merged the PBL with the traditional curriculum. The principles set forth by this group are seeing their full fruition in the current curriculum with an emphasis on small group interaction and a sharp curtailment of lectures and total contact time to allow students more time for reflection and problem solving. His Medical Clerkship cardiology skills modules recognize the new role of physical diagnosis required to compliment modern imaging technology and have provided students with the practical skills that will enable them to provide adequate care to patients with cardiovascular disease in a primary care setting. Throughout his career he has been a staunch advocate for the primary prevention of heart disease. He established the HVI Lipid Clinic for complex lipoprotein problems during his last decade on the faculty. Dr. Zelis looks back on his career in Hershey with pride and satisfaction and feels that his move here was an excellent one for both him and his family.

DEPARTMENT of MEDICINE, DIVISION of CLINICAL PHARMACOLOGY -- ARTHUR H(ull) HAYES, M.D.; founding Chief, 1972-81. Hayes was born July 18, 1933 in Highland Park, MI (died February 11, 2010). He received his A.B. in Philosophy, *magna cum laude* from Santa Clara University, CA in 1955, and then went to Oxford University, England as a Rhodes Scholar, earning a doctorate in philosophy, politics, and economics in 1957. He returned to the US to study medicine, first at Georgetown University Medical School and graduated from Cornell University Medical School in 1964. He served in the United States Army Medical Corps from 1965-67, achieving the rank of Captain.

Hayes started his academic career at Cornell University Medical School in 1967 as an Assistant Professor of Medicine and Pharmacology and Associate Dean for Academic Programs. In 1970, Hayes and his wife co-founded a medical clinic on the Pacific island Pohnpei, and they worked as a physician-nurse team on behalf of the Jesuit Missions. He was appointed as Associate Professor of Medicine and Pharmacology and Chief of Clinical Pharmacology at TMSHMC in 1972. He was later promoted to Professor.

Hayes was appointed Commissioner of the Food and Drug Administration (FDA) by President Ronald Reagan in 1981. During his years at the agency, he directed the FDA's response to the Tylenol tampering cases, called for a voluntary moratorium on direct-to-consumer advertising of prescription medicines, and weathered criticism on the FDA's approval of the sweetener aspartame.

After leaving the FDA, Hayes served as Provost and Dean at the New York Medical College and later, in 1986 was appointed

President of E M Pharmaceuticals. Five years later, he founded MediScience Associates and retired in 2005.

Hayes served on numerous boards, received many honorary degrees and awards and was named a Visiting Professor at several academic institutions. He authored more than 100 professional papers and trained many clinical pharmacologists.

DEPARTMENT of MEDICINE, DIVISION of EMERGENCY MEDICINE -- H. ARNOLD MULLER, M.D.

Dr. Muller was appointed as the founding Chief of the Division of Emergency Medicine in 1973, as an Assistant Professor, and promoted to Associate Professor in 1978.

He was born April 16, 1930 in Albany, NY. He attended Dartmouth College (1948-52) and received an A.B., Biology-Chemistry (*cum laude*) and was Phi Beta Kappa. He was accepted by the Dartmouth Medical School (1951-53) after 3 years of undergraduate study. At that time, Dartmouth only had the first two years of medical school, and he completed his studies at Harvard Medical School, receiving the M.D. in 1955.

Muller did his internship at the Pennsylvania Hospital, Philadelphia, PA. Since he did not receive a salary or stipend as an intern, he joined the U.S. Air Force for financial support. He continued to be supported by the Air Force through his medical residency at the University of Washington, Seattle, WA. After his residency, he had military pay back time. He served first as Chief of Medicine at Tyndall Air Force Base, FL (1959-64) and then at Westover Air Force Base, MA. He was seriously considering a career in the Air Force when he learned of an internal medicine practice in Carlisle, PA. He left that practice in 1973 to develop the Emergency Medicine Division at TMSHMC. Prior to that time emergency rooms were primarily run by medicine and surgery residents. His vision was to establish Emergency Medicine as a specialty of medicine. In 1979, he took a leave of absence from the faculty to serve as Secretary of Health, Commonwealth of Pennsylvania. After his government service, in 1987 he served as Chief of Staff, Veterans

Administration, Lebanon, PA and returned part time as Professor of Emergency Medicine, TMSHMC.

Muller loved the practice of medicine, and always worked part time in other clinics in addition to his regular job. He played a major role in establishing Emergency Medicine as a specialty and served as President of the American College of Emergency Medicine.

DEPARTMENT of MEDICINE, DIVISION of ENDOCRINOLOGY -- C. WAYNE BARDIN; M.D.

Dr Bardin was appointed as the founding Chief of the Division of Endocrinology in 1970 as an Associate Professor, and promoted to Professor in 1972. He was born in West Texas and received his B.A. (Biology) from Rice University in 1957. He received his M.S (Biology with honor) and M.D. (with honor) in 1962 from Baylor University. He also completed all of the courses and research for a PhD but did not meet all of the time requirements. However, he did receive Doctor *Honoris Causa* degrees from the University of Caen, France (1990), University of Pierre and Marie Curie, France (1996), and the University of Helsinki, Finland (2000).

Dr. Bardin did his internship and residency at the New York Hospital-Cornell Medical Center (1962-64); then transferred to the Endocrinology Branch, NCI, NIH (1964-70), with specialization in Internal Medicine and Endocrinology. He had a very successful career at the NIH studying reproductive endocrinology and cancer. However, he began to wonder about his future career development; i.e. scientific pursuit or academic leadership.

He developed a strong research program at Hershey but realized that he could not successfully pursue academic leadership and scientific investigation on the scale that he envisioned. He chose the latter but there was insufficient research space to grow his program. In 1979 Bardin was offered, and accepted the position as Vice President of the Population Council and Director of the Center for Biomedical Research at the Rockefeller University, New York, NY. This enabled him to develop a large, multi-national research program for the multiple drug delivery systems for use in reproductive health care and cancer treatment. His primary research focus was to determine how hormones regulate human genes, and developed products for reproductive health care and cancer therapy. He directed basic and clinical research leading to over 500 scientific publications and patents.

He was appointed to the editorial boards of 15 journals. He also served on national and international committees and boards for NIH, WHO, the Ford Foundation, Rockefeller Foundation, and numerous scientific societies. He received many honors and awards for his contributions and accomplishments.

DEPARTMENT of MEDICINE, DIVISION of ENDOCRINOLOGY – Richard J. Santen, M.D.

Dr. Santen was born April 2, 1939 in Cincinnati, OH. He attended Catholic grade and high school. His father urged him to go to Yale for his undergraduate studies, but one of the Jesuit priests said no, he should get a good Jesuit education to learn to think more clearly and logically. So he chose Holy Cross College (A.B., 1961). He majored in Philosophy because he thought the liberal arts education was probably better preparation for medical school than focusing intensively on science. He received his M.D. degree from the University of Michigan, Ann Harbor, MI in 1965.

He did his internship in medicine at New York Hospital, Cornell Medical Center, NY (1965-66) He remained there as an Assistant Resident (1966-67), then transferred to the University Hospital, Ann Arbor, MI as a Senior Resident (1967-69). He joined the U.S.P.H.S. (Berry Plan) and was simultaneously an Endocrinology Fellow, University of Washington, Seattle, WA (1969-71).

He began his academic career as an Assistant Professor of Medicine, TMSHMC in 1971, promoted to Associate Professor in 1975, and to Professor in 1979. He was attracted to Hershey because of Wayne Bardin. They had similar research interests and Bardin was a rising star in the field of Endocrinology. Dr. Santen was named an Evan Pugh Professor of Medicine in 1986. He was named Chief of Endocrinology in 1979, and served as Vice Chair of Medicine (1992-93). During his time at Hershey, he had two sabbaticals; Visiting Professor, University of Liege, Liege, Belgium (1978-79), and Visiting Professor, Hospital Necker, Paris, France (1985-86).

He left Hershey in 1993 to serve as Professor and Chairman of Medicine, Wayne State University, Detroit, MI (1993-95), and Interim Director, Meyer L. Prentis Comprehensive Cancer Center of Metropolitan Detroit, Michigan Cancer Foundation, Detroit, MI. In 1995, he was named Professor of Medicine, Division of Endocrinology and Metabolism, University of Virginia, Charlottesville, VA.

DEPARTMENT of MEDICINE, DIVISION of HEMATOLOGY and ONCOLOGY -- DAVID E. JENKINS, Jr M.D.

Dr. Jenkins was the founding Division Chief (1970-73). He was born June 3. 1932 in Niles, OH. Jenkins received his A.B. (Psychology) in 1954 from Yale University, and M.D. (1958) from the School of Medicine, Western Reserve University, Cleveland, OH in 1958. He completed Postgraduate training as an Intern (Internal Medicine), 1958-59, at New York Hospital, Cornell Medical Center; Assistant Resident (Internal Medicine), 1959-61, and Hematology Research Fellow, 1961-63, at the same institution.

Dr. Jenkins began his academic career in 1963 as Chief of Hematology, Nashville Veterans Medical Center and Instructor of Medicine at Vanderbilt University, Nashville, TN. He was promoted to Assistant Professor in 1965, and to Associate Professor in 1968. In the late 1960's he was asked to consider positions in Hematology at several medical centers along with positions in Transfusion Medicine because of his expertise in red cell immunology. Eventually, he was recruited to TMSHMC in 1970 as Associate Professor of Medicine and Chief, Division of Hematology, and promoted in 1971 to Professor of Medicine and Chief, Division of Hematology and Oncology. He was the second full time clinical academic faculty to arrive at TMSHMC and he worked very closely with Dr. Graham Jeffries (Chair of Medicine) to coordinate clinical teaching programs during that academic year and in the development of the Department of

Medicine from 1970-73. In 1973, he turned his professional focus to Transfusion Medicine when he was recruited to return to Nashville as Director, American Red Cross Blood Services, Nashville Region and Medical Director, Vanderbilt Medical Center Transfusion Service with academic appointments as Professor of Medicine, Vanderbilt (1973-81), and Professor of Medicine and Pathology (1980-81). From 1981-86, he served as President, CEO and Medical Director of the Central Blood Bank of Pittsburgh and Professor of Pathology and Medicine at the University of Pittsburgh. He then went to the School of Medicine, University of California, San Francisco as Professor of Medicine in Residence and Assistant Dean. In 1988, he was recruited to serve as Director, American Red Cross Blood Services, Louisville (KY) Region with an academic appointment as Clinical Professor of Pathology and Medicine at the University of Louisville (1988-2002). He is a Diplomate of the American Board of Internal Medicine (Internal Medicine- 1968 and Hematology-1972), and the American Board of Pathology, Blood Banking/Transfusion Medicine (1976).

Dr. Jenkins returned to TMSHMC in 2002 as Clinical Professor of Medicine and Pathology and has served as a volunteer faculty member since that time. He has/had been active in a number of Professional and Scientific Societies (24), University and Hospital Committees and Offices (30), Local, State and National Committees (22).

He has received 5 research grants with a focus on antibody and complement and red cell interactions, hemolytic anemia, and Paroxysmal Nocturnal Hemoglobinuria. He has served as an Editorial Reviewer for 5 medical journals and has published 46 scientific articles in peer reviewed journals.

DEPARTMENT of MEDICINE, DIVISION of HEMATOLOGY – M. ELAINE EYSTER, A.B., M.D.

Dr. Eyster was born March 21, 1935 in York, PA. She received her A.B. from Duke University (*magna cum laude*,1956), and M.D. from the same institution in 1961. She was initially interested in Bucknell for her undergraduate studies, but her father persuaded her to go to Duke. She majored in chemistry and minored in math. She favored the sciences over the arts because they seemed to be more logical. Her original goal was to be a chemist. However she decided that she liked biology better, and would try to work to find solutions to health related problems, and work with people rather than molecules. She chose Duke for medical school because she felt very comfortable there as an undergraduate. A close friend of hers was a year ahead of her in medical school. The friend had gone to Cornell/New York Hospital in Pediatrics. Eyster followed her to take a few electives. She felt comfortable there, and applied for a residency in Medicine, and completed it in 1963. This was followed by an NIH Fellowship (1963-66). After her fellowship, she was appointed Assistant Professor of Medicine, Cornell University (1967-70).

She was recruited to TMSHMC as an Assistant Professor of Medicine in the Division of Hematology in 1970, promoted to Associate Professor in 1973, and to Professor in 1982. Over the intervening years Dr. Eyster has made many important contributions to the Medical Center and to her specialty. These accomplishments have been recognized locally, nationally, and internationally. She was appointed Chief, Division of Hematology (1973-96). When state funding became available in 1973 she established the Central Pennsylvania Hemophilia Center. She has served as Director of that program since that time. A key factor in the success of the Hemophilia Program has been the Special Hematology/Hemostasis Laboratory which was founded by Dr. Eyster to support the Hemophilia Program. From these bases she has made many important contributions to the understanding of bleeding and clotting disorders. She has also made important contributions to the improved treatment of patients with bleeding and clotting disorders and has published extensively on her areas of expertise.

One of the tragic complications for hemophilia patients in the 1970's and early 1980's was the development of post transfusion hepatitis and HIV. Dr. Eyster became an important contributor to the development of methods for treating these complications and, more important, to understand them and treat them. She and her co-workers participated in crucial clinical trials of new and improved coagulation factors of higher purity and safety to eliminate those risks. She has published extensively on these observations. Because of the recognized quality of her scientific work she has continuously maintained a high level of extramural funding throughout her career. Along with these impressive scientific and service accomplishments she has maintained a dedicated and effective teacher, and remains very active in the teaching of medical students, residents, trainees, and professional colleagues.

Dr. Eyster was promoted to Associate Professor in 1973, and to Professor in 1982. She has held the academic rank of Distinguished Professor of Medicine since 1991 as well as a joint appointment as Professor of Pathology since 1998.

DEPARTMENT of MEDICINE, DIVISION OF INTERNAL MEDICINE -- JOHN BURNSIDE, M.D.

Dr. Burnside was born January 15, 1941 in Pennsylvania, then moved to IL as a teenager when his father's job was transferred. He cites his oldest brother as having a significant influence on him. His oldest brother was a veterinary student (UP) and commuted from home. He recalled reading his books, especially anatomy. He enrolled in the University of Illinois, Champaign, IL. Since he knew he wanted to be a physician, he transferred to the medical school in Chicago (MD with Very High Honors, 1966). He was encouraged to apply to the Massachusetts General Hospital, Boston, MA. To his surprise, he was accepted and went there for his internship (1966-67) and residency. In between being an Assistant Resident (1967-68) and Resident in Medicine (1969-70) he chose to do a year as an Assistant Resident in Pathology (1968-69) because he wanted to "see things from the inside". He then served as Clinical Research Fellow (1970) and Chief Resident in Medicine (1971).

His primary goal was general internal medicine working with patients and teaching medical students and residents. He had heard about TMSHMC and contacted the Chair of Medicine (Dr. Graham Jeffries) to see if there might be a spot for him in the department as a general internist seeing patients and teaching. Jeffries had a similar vision, but suggested that he be the Head of the Division of Internal Medicine. He was the only person in the division but, as the patient care and teaching rapidly increased he was able to recruit Drs. Trautlein, Kammerer, and McGlynn.

The successor Dean (Prystowsky) recognized Burnside's talents, and quickly asked him to serve in a variety of administrative roles. In addition to his position as Chief of Internal Medicine, he served as Director of Ambulatory Services; Vice Chair, Center for Humanistic Studies; Vice Chair of Medicine; Associate Dean for Patient Care; and Associate Provost and Dean for Health Affairs. During that time, he also served as Acting Chair of Medicine (1983) and two terms as Acting Senior Vice President for Health Affairs and Dean (1983 and 1986-87). He describes these administrative appointments as being a problem solver, reflecting his strengths as a good number two man. However, his clinical passion was the care and treatment of patients.

He left in 1987 to be Associate Dean at the Southwestern Medical Center, The University of Texas, Dallas, TX. He spent the next 13 years working on the enhancement of Clinical Programs at Southwestern, including the building of a new hospital. Since his retirement in 2000, he and his wife have run a horse ranch which they enjoy doing very much. In addition, he has served as an active clinical consultant to a number of institutions in Texas on a part time basis in his retirement.

DEPARTMENT of MEDICINE, DIVISION of ONCOLOGY – ALLAN LIPTON, M.D.

Dr. Lipton was born in Brooklyn, NY in 1937. He received his undergraduate degree from Amherst College and his M.D. degree from New York University. While at NYU, he had contact with many outstanding scientists on the faculty who stimulated his interest in pursuing a research career. Following graduation, he completed two years of residency in Internal Medicine in the Cornell (Second) Division of Bellevue Hospital which included four months rotation at Memorial Sloan-Kettering which provided an early exposure to oncology. After two years of residency he received an appointment as a Research Associate with Dr. Arthur Weissbach, a biochemist at the National Institute of Allergy and Infectious Diseases, NIH. During this time he did basic research on nucleic acids and bacteriophages. After NIH he completed his clinical training with two years of fellowship in hematology-oncology at Memorial Sloan-Kettering and New York Hospital where he was exposed to an outstanding group of leaders who were on the Memorial staff at that time. After Memorial Sloan-Kettering he spent two years in San Diego as an American Cancer Society Dernham Fellow at the Salk Institute studying growth factors in the laboratory of Dr. Robert Holley, who had won the Nobel Prize in 1968 for his work on isolating and determining the structure of transfer-RNA.

At the completion of his fellowship in 1971, Dr. Lipton was asked to look at faculty positions at several medical centers in the US. He chose Hershey, in part, because he was intrigued by the challenge of starting a new program in a new institution. From 1971-73 he served as a member of the Division of Hematology/Oncology. In 1973, the Division of Oncology was established as a separate Division and Lipton was appointed as Chief. He held that position until 1996 when Hematology/Oncology was combined, once again, as a part of the process to establish the Cancer Institute which opened in 2009.

Throughout his career in Hershey Dr. Lipton has been a dedicated and productive clinical investigator. His program has always been well funded from a variety of sources. He has had extensive and productive collaborations with other faculty members from the Department of Medicine as well as other Medical Center Departments. The collaboration between the Division of Oncology, Dr. Richard Santen of the Division of Endocrinology and Dr. Larry Demers in Pathology has been very strong, particularly in studies related to the role of aromatase inhibitors in the treatment of carcinoma of the breast.

Dr. Lipton was appointed as an Assistant Professor of Medicine in 1971. He was promoted to Associate Professor in 1974, and Professor of Medicine in 1979. Dr. Lipton looks back on his years in Hershey with great fondness and appreciation. He believes he has been able to achieve many important personal goals and is deeply appreciative of his interactions with and support from so many excellent colleagues.

DEPARTMENT of OBSTETRICS and GYNECOLOGY --

VINCENT G STENGER, M.D., founding Chair, 1970-78. He was born January 27, 1932 in Wheeling, West Virginia. He received his B.S. from West Liberty State College, WV in 1954. He was raised on a farm in West Virginia, and had originally planned to be a veterinarian. However, an uncle, who was in family practice, encouraged him to go to medical school. He applied to the Johns Hopkins University School of Medicine (JHUSM). At that time, interviews were conducted by former graduates who lived in the area of the applicant. After his acceptance, an uncle drove him to the JHUSM; it was his first visit to Baltimore and the JHUSM. He received his M.D. degree in 1958.

In medical school, he found the first 2 years to be difficult with mid-term Anatomy exams and trying to stay awake in the Pathology slide shows. However, he found the clinical years were exciting and fun. He loved Medicine, Surgery, Obstetrics, Gynecology, Pediatrics, and Ophthalmology, but was somewhat cool on Psychiatry. Psychiatry was a 4 week clinical outpatient rotation. After one week, he and two other students drove to Ft Lauderdale and spent two weeks partying with college students.

Stenger went to the University of Florida (Gainesville, FL), Department of Obstetrics & Gynecology first as Chief Resident and Instructor (1961), then Instructor (1962-63), Assistant Professor (1963-67), and Associate Professor (1967-70) Department of Obstetrics & Gynecology as well as Department of Pharmacology & Therapeutics (1967-69).

He was recruited to TMSHMC in 1970 as Professor and Chairman of Obstetrics & Gynecology. He left in 1978 for private practice in FL, first in a group practice, then solo as the other members of the group retired. He is currently the sole practitioner of the Sarasota Life Extension Institute, practicing age preventive medicine,

At the University of Florida, he established a basic science research program using a breeding colony of monkeys (*Macaca arctoides*) to study menstrual cycles and breeding/ovulation timing, and sampling of fetal blood *in utero* based on bilobate placenta. He moved the entire colony of monkeys to Hershey and continued his studies on fetal liver metabolism. He has 60 publications on basic and clinical studies in peer reviewed journals. He found the recruitment of research oriented faculty to be difficult. He went to national meetings and listened to their scientific presentations. In retrospect, he believes that he was not aggressive enough for successful recruitment.

DEPARTMENT of OBSTETRICS and GYNECOLOGY, DIVISION of GYNECOLOGIC ONCOLOGY -- RODRIQUE MORTEL, M.D. founding Chief, 1972.

Born on December 3, 1933 in Saint Marc, Haiti, Dr. Mortel has published his autobiography (*I AM FROM HAITI*, 2000, The Mortel Family Charitable Foundation, P.O. Box 405, Hershey, PA 17033) covering the period from his childhood, through secondary, undergraduate, medical school, and residency training; and early experiences, first as Chief of Gynecologic Oncology, then Chairman of the Department of Obstetrics & Gynecology, and later as the Director of the Penn State Cancer Center.

As detailed in his autobiography, Dr. Mortel was a man of strong determination and crucial timing. Education, drive, ambition, and a strong religious faith were the guidelines for his life's plan. Raised in poverty, and often hungry, he realized that an education was the only way out of this despair. However, living in a country with an 85 % illiteracy rate (the highest in the western hemisphere), this challenge was almost insurmountable; and it was only through sheer determination that he and his mother were able to achieve their goals. No matter what he did, it was always with the determination to be "the best".

Dr. Mortel, in 1954, began his six-year journey of studies at Haiti's Port-au-Prince Medical School. He was always in the top 5 of his medical school class, and graduated *magna cum laude* in

1960. The government had decreed that his graduating class would serve two years in rural clinics as government physicians. After he completed his government service, he went to the Hospital de la Misericorde in Montreal, Canada in 1962. He chose the specialty of Obstetrics & Gynecology because it was then the only one available in that hospital. In 1963, he accepted an offer of an internship at the Mercy-Douglass Hospital in Philadelphia, PA. In 1965, he accepted a residency in Obstetrics & Gynecology at the Hahnemann Medical College in Philadelphia.

His Chief at Hahnemann strongly encouraged him to consider the subspecialty of Gynecologic Oncology. He realized this would enable him to be not only a clinician, but also a teacher and a researcher. In 1969, he began fellowship training at the Memorial Sloan-Kettering Cancer Center in New York City. At the end of his fellowship he returned to Hahnemann Medical College and Hospital as a senior instructor in the Department of Obstetrics & Gynecology (1970). The next year (1971), he was promoted to Assistant Professor in the new Division of Gynecologic Oncology at Hahnemann.

In 1972, Dr. Mortel was invited to join TMSHMC and develop a program in gynecologic oncology. He had been recommended by the Chief at Memorial Sloan-Kettering. He saw this as an opportunity to design and develop a strong program in gynecologic oncology, combining patient care, teaching, and basic research; and where faculty and fellows would be provided protected time for clinical and/or basic research.

He took a sabbatical leave (1978-79) to study hormone dependence of endometrial carcinoma at the Department de Chimie Biologique at the Universite de Paris XI. During that time, Mortel was also asked to design, develop, and establish a special program for the University of Paris. He was also offered a new position in research and clinical practice, combining the services of 4 institutions: Sloan-Kettering Institute, Memorial Hospital, Cornell University, and Rockefeller University in New York City. He was invited to interview for the Directorship at the Curie Institute in Paris, France. He decided to accept the offer in New York City but was obligated to return to TMSHMC for two years in return for his sabbatical year. He returned, but planned to return to Paris, France to continue his research with the Ligue Nationale Francaise Contre le Cancer. During the year back at TMSHMC, he was the Acting Chair of Obstetrics & Gynecology, when Dr. Chez resigned. He was asked several times to apply for the permanent Chair, but refused. In the previous 2 years, the department had fallen apart, and he was being asked to re-build it. Finally, he agreed to accept the challenge. He did so in a superb manner.

In 1985, Dr. Mortel accepted a new position to plan and establish a cancer center to match the overall high quality of TMSHMC. His goal was to build a cancer center without walls in which all elements would work together but not necessarily be housed together. In 1995, he was formally appointed Associate Dean and Director of the Penn State Cancer Center.

Dr. Mortel received many honors and awards, including the Horatio Alger Award and Robert Wood Johnson Policy Fellow Award.

Throughout the years, Mortel always had an abiding love and depth of caring for the country of his birth. Although he made many contributions to his country, his most recent is the building of 4 schools in Haiti; Les Bons Samaritains elementary school, the James Stine High School, a trade school, and a literacy school.

DEPARTMENT of PATHOLOGY -- RICHARD L. NAEYE, MD; founding Chair, 1967

Dr. Richard L. Naeye was born November 27, 1929 in Rochester, NY. His father's family were Dutch immigrants who settled in a very fertile, rural area of New York. His father was the first person in the community to graduate from college, and the community made him president of their canning factory. Naeye's youth was spent attending the local, small schools, and working in the vegetable fields for the canning factory. His parents strongly encouraged him and his brother towards higher education.

He graduated from Colgate University in 1951 (A.B.) and Columbia University in 1955 (M.D.). He received scholarships to both universities, based on competitive examinations.

Naeye aspired to be a physician from an early age, but was more interested in clinical research than community service. He believed that he would have greater opportunities for clinical research as a pathologist. After graduation from medical school, he did an internship in internal medicine (1955-56) so he could be certified to practice medicine. He then completed a residency (1956-58) in pathology at Columbia-Presbyterian Medical Center, New York City, NY. He continued his training in pathology at the University of Vermont College of Medicine, Burlington, VT (1960-63). He is board certified in both anatomic and clinical pathology.

He started his academic career as an Assistant Professor of Pathology at the University of Vermont College of Medicine in 1960, and was promoted to Associate Professor in 1963, and to Professor in 1967. He was a Markle Scholar in Academic Medicine (1960-65). This award enabled him to develop his clinical research at a relatively early age. He was appointed Professor and Chairman, Department of Pathology, College of Medicine, TPSU in 1967. He served in that capacity until 1997 when he gave up the chairmanship to devote more time to his clinical research activities. He was honored by his appointment as University Professor of Pathology in 1984.

Naeye's research centered on the effects of disease on society, with a particular emphasis on placental pathology. He was a member of many societies related to his areas of expertise. He was an active contributor to the scientific literature with over 250 publications.

He retired in 2005. In retirement, he devoted his time to nature photography. He was a strong advocate of using photography to "really see" the beauty around us.

Dr Naeye passed away December 10, 2013.

DEPARTMENT of PATHOLOGY, DIVISION of ANATOMIC PATHOLOGY -- ARTHUR ABT, M. D.

Dr. Abt was born May 28, 1940 in Newark, NJ. His mother was a school teacher and his father a textile engineer. He became interested in medicine as a child and may have developed an interest in Pathology because the father of a good friend was a Pathologist. He attended public schools in Newark, NJ. He was a pre-med major in a highly competitive program at Rutgers University, New Brunswick, NJ, receiving a B.A. in 1962. He then enrolled in the George Washington University, Washington, D.C. and received his M.D.degree in 1966. Although he knew that he wanted to specialize in pathology, he did an internship in medicine (George Washington University Hospital) because he thought that it would help him to better understand the pathology services being requested by the referring clinicians. He did his residency in Pathology at the Mt. Sinai School of Medicine in New York, NY. Although he knew that he wanted to specialize in Surgical Pathology, he fulfilled the requirements for certification in both anatomic and clinical pathology. He fulfilled his military service obligation in the U.S.P.H.S. in the Department of Pathology, U.S.P.H.S. Hospital, Baltimore, MD (1971-73).

He was appointed to the faculty of TMSHMC as an Assistant Professor in 1973 as a member of the Division of Anatomic Pathology headed by Dr. Malcom McGavran. After McGavran left Hershey, Abt served as Acting Chief of Anatomic Pathology from 1976-78. In 1978 he was appointed as permanent Chief of Anatomic Pathology. He was promoted to Associate Professor (1977-82) and Professor in 1982. He served as Chief of the Division of Anatomic Pathology (1978-97). He was Vice Chair of the Department of Pathology (1994-97) and Chairman of Pathology from 1997 to 2002. Under Dr. Abt's leadership the Anatomic Pathology Division grew and provided strong support for both patient services and faculty research programs. In his own research Dr. Abt collaborated extensively with other Medical Center faculty bringing his expertise in anatomic pathology to enhance their research.

He served, with distinction, on many medical center and university committees. He feels his most important contributions were made as chair of the Curriculum Committee.

DEPARTMENT of PATHOLOGY, DIVISION of CLINICAL PATHOLOGY -- ARTHUR F.KRIEG, M.D., founding Chief (1968-96). Krieg was born October 23, 1930 in East Orange, NJ. He received his AB. (Psychology) from Yale in 1952, and his M.D. degree from Tufts University in 1956. He was a rotating intern (1956-57) and resident in pathology under Dr. Alan R. Moritz (1957-60) at University Hospitals in Cleveland, OH. He then served in the USAF (Berry Plan, 1960-62). Upon his discharge, he completed his residency in clinical pathology under Bradley E. Copeland (1962-64) at the New England Deaconess Hospital in Boston, MA.

His original career goal was to be an engineer, following in his father's footsteps. However, he thoroughly enjoyed his liberal arts classes in psychology, intellectual history, English, and philosophy. He changed his major to Liberal Arts (psychology), but took enough chemistry courses so he could go to graduate school in chemical engineering. In his senior year at Yale he applied to graduate school; University of Washington for psychology and neurology and MIT for chemical engineering. However, he also applied to medical school and, in retrospect, feels this was a good decision. He attended Tufts University School of Medicine in Boston, MA and graduated in 1956.

Krieg began his academic career as an Assistant Professor of Pathology at the State University of New York, Upstate Medical Center, Syracuse, NY (1964-68). They were building a new hospital, and he was in charge of establishing a new clinical chemistry laboratory. His duties expanded to other areas including hematology and blood banking. He realized the potential of computers to handle clinical laboratory data and worked with the Department of Computer Science at the University of Syracuse, and to make this a reality. This came to the attention of Dr. Naeye (founding chair of Pathology) who recruited him to Hershey. He has published widely, received many honors and citations, and is recognized as one of the prominent leaders in development of laboratory information systems.

DEPARTMENT of PATHOLOGY, DIVISION of CLINICAL PATHOLOGY--LAURENCE M. DEMERS, Ph.D., DABBC, FACB

Dr. Demers is Distinguished Professor Emeritus of Pathology and Medicine. He was the Founding Director of Clinical Chemistry and the Core Endocrine Laboratory.

He is a graduate of Merrimack College in North Andover, MA, and received his doctorate in biochemistry from the State University of New York, Upstate Medical Center, Syracuse, in 1970. He completed a post-doctoral fellowship in Biochemical Endocrinology at Harvard Medical School, and after one year as an instructor at Harvard left in 1973 to accept a position as Assistant Professor of Pathology at the newly created Penn State University College of Medicine. He was awarded the title of full Professor in 1982, and in 1997 was given the title of Distinguished Professor of Pathology by the President of Penn State University. In 1982, he received an NIH Fogarty Senior International Fellowship for the study of hypertension in pregnancy at the University of Oxford, UK.

Dr. Demers is a diplomat of the American Board of Clinical Chemistry and a Fellow of the National Academy of Clinical Biochemistry. He has been active in clinical laboratory medicine at the local, state, and national levels. He served as Chairman of the Technical Advisory Committee to the state of PA, Department of Health from 1984-92. He has been active nationally with the American Association of Clinical Chemistry (AACC), having served as a member of the Clinical Chemistry Journal editorial board for over 10 years and 5 years as its editorial editor. He served on the AACC Board of Directors, both as an at large member (1992-94) and as President and Chairman of the Board in 1997. He served as Chair (1997-2007) of the Van Slyke Society, the philanthropic arm of the AACC.

He served as Secretary (1984) and President (1981) of the National Academy of Clinical Biochemistry. He also served on the Board of Directors of the Clinical Ligand Assay Society from 1995-97. Demers has served on the editorial boards of nine journals, and has membership in nine societies.

Demers has carried out extensive research program with grant support from the NIH, pharmaceutical companies, diagnostic companies, and foundations, exceeding $8 million in direct costs. His research in breast cancer, metastatic bone disease, steroid metabolism, and lung disease has resulted in over 743 publications, including 7 books and 57 book chapters.

Dr Demers has been the recipient of numerous awards. In 1971, he received the Lalor Foundation Award for his work in reproductive endocrinology at Harvard Medical School. In 1974, he was awarded a Pharmaceutical Manufacturers Association First award for his work on bile acids and liver disease. In 1982, he received an NIH Senior Fogarty Award for study at the University of Oxford in England. In 1986, he was the 35th recipient of the Bayer (Siemens) award given by the AACC for outstanding contributions to Clinical Chemistry. In 1991, he received the Alvin Dubin award from the National Academy of Biochemistry for service to the profession of clinical biochemistry. More recently he received the Morton K. Schwartz award from the AACC for significant accomplishment in Cancer Diagnostics in July, 2010 for his contributions to Cancer Research Diagnostics.

Demers served on the Board of Trustees at Merrimack College, North Andover, MA from 2000 to 2010 and was Chairman of the Board for the last three of those years.

DEPARTMENT of PATHOLOGY, DIVISION OF EXPERIMENTAL PATHOLOGY, JOHN W. KREIDER, M.D., founding Chief, 1975-97. Kreider was born in 1938 (died January 29, 2010). He received a B.A. in Biology from LaSalle College in 1959, and his M.D. degree from the University of Pennsylvania School of Medicine in 1963. He interned at Yale University (1963-64), and completed his postdoctoral fellowship in pathology at the University of Pennsylvania Medical School, Department of Pathology in 1967.

Kreider was given joint appointments in the Departments of Pathology and Microbiology as an Assistant Professor in 1967 and subsequently promoted to Associate Professor and Professor. He served as Chief of Experimental Pathology, 1975-97. He was a founding member of the Jake Gittlen Cancer Research Institute in 1970 and served as Director, concurrently with his other academic responsibilities. Kreider, in conjunction with Warren Gittlen, developed a unique funding source, in memory of Warren's father, to establish the Institute; raising over $14 million for research.

Kreider was a talented writer, speaker and communicator, both among his peers in the scientific community and with the general public. He had a favorite saying "if you can't explain your science to the public, then you don't understand it yourself".

Kreider's research specialized in the study of human papilloma viruses, one of the leading causes of cervical cancer in women. He received countless research grants from federal and private agencies and held numerous patents with his long-term collaborator in the Department of Microbiology, Mary K. Howett, Ph.D. Their work led to the discovery of a method for propagating human papilloma viruses which, in turn, contributed to the development of the HPV vaccine, Gardasil, released by Merck Pharmaceutical Company in 2006. He was the author of more than 150 publications in peer reviewed journals.

Kreider's teaching style was greatly appreciated by the students. He received the Teaching Excellence Award, given by the second year medical students, 11 times between 1980 and 1990. He was awarded The Pennsylvania State University Faculty Scholar Medal for Outstanding Achievement in Health and Life Sciences in 1990.

Kreider was an enthusiastic outdoorsman, and served as a volunteer Deputy Game Protector for the Pennsylvania Game Commission (primarily so he could trap cottontail rabbits as a source of virus material). Of course, some still remember the time he tried to roast a wild turkey in the department's autoclave.

In his retirement years, he was free to pursue his lifelong interest in model railroading. His home-based business, Father Nature, produced highly realistic model trees and were highly prized by hobbyists.

DEPARTMENT of PEDIATRICS -- NICHOLAS M(acy) NELSON; founding Chair, 1970-89, and continuing as Professor of Pediatrics until his retirement in 1998.

Dr. Nelson was born in Baltimore, MD (6/11/29) and died in Topsham, ME (1/26/14). He was raised in New Brunswick, NJ, and graduated from Deerfield Academy (1946), Yale University (B.S., 1950), and Cornell University Medical College (M.D., 1954).

He majored in zoology and minored in chemistry at Yale, planning to continue his studies in Graduate School. He was particularly interested in spiders, and anticipated a career in arachnoidology. He spent the summer between his college junior and senior years as a circulating nurse at St. Luke's Hospital in New York City. About this time he began to consider a career in medicine. Having majored in zoology, he did not have courses to make up to be eligible to apply to medical school.

He and a classmate from Deerfield Academy applied to McGill, University of Pennsylvania, and Harvard. They were accepted by all three, and turned down all three. They had also applied to Cornell and Columbia. Nelson went to Cornell and his friend to Columbia.

Nelson did an internship (Medicine) and started his residency (Medicine) at Bellevue Hospital in New York City. After three months in Medicine, he converted to Pediatrics.

He served in the U.S. Army Medical Corps (Berry Plan) in France (1956-58). Upon completion of his military service, he became Senior Assistant Resident at Children's Hospital Medical Center in Boston, MA. He then accepted a Fellowship at the Boston Lying-in Hospital under the supervision of Dr. Clement Smith, considered by many as the father of neonatology.

Nelson went into private practice with an older pediatrician in New Brunswick, NJ. After 2 ½ years, he decided to return to academia to work with Dr. Clement Smith, ultimately becoming Director of Smith's service. He also became an Associate Editor of the New England Journal of Medicine, and received a competitive Research Career Development Award (RCDA) from the NIH.

In 1970, he started looking for a job because Dr. Smith was retiring. He was being recruited by Washington University in St. Louis, MO but was having second thoughts about the position, primarily because the landscape was so different from his native NJ.

Dr. Harrell (founding Dean of TMSHMC) called Nelson to ask if he was interested in being considered as chair of Pediatrics at the new College of Medicine. Dr. Nelson's vision in accepting the position was to expand his passion for research and education in neonatology. He knew that it would be difficult because neonatology was a new field, the Teaching Hospital was still under construction, and the College of Medicine had yet to make its mark.

Nelson did not find recruiting faculty to be particularly difficult. He did not personally know most of his recruits; however, he did rely heavily on recommendations from people with whom he had worked, or knew personally. His biggest problem was adequate space for young faculty trying to establish their research programs. Another deterrent was the lack of an identifiable Children's Hospital. Most of his recruits had trained in Children's Hospitals at other institutions. He was able to renovate adjacent space for clinical activities, but that was neither ideal nor adequate. He laid the ground work for a Children's Hospital, which only became a reality after he retired.

He encouraged his faculty to develop research programs. He did not care what the focus of their research would be but it had to be related to their specialty and of high quality. Several recruits mentioned that he appeared to select faculty on the basis of who they were rather than to fill a job.

Dr. Nelson emphasized pediatric education to both medical students and residents. He found this to be challenging because of the size of his faculty, and the lack of a critical mass in some areas. He judged the education efforts of his department to be about average compared to other programs, but viewed it as being on an upward trajectory when he retired.

Dr. Nelson thoroughly enjoyed the written word, and throughout his career, authored and edited many medical articles, journals, and textbooks. His textbook on neonatology, written jointly with his mentor (Dr, Clement Smith), is considered a classic in the field.

DIVISION of GENERAL PEDIATRICS, DEPARTMENT of PEDIATRICS -- CHESTON M(ilton) BERLIN, JR, M.D., Founding Chief (1984-2000). He was born March 28, 1936 in Pittsburgh, PA. He graduated from the Mt. Lebanon High School in Pittsburgh.

His mother was a nurse, and he often read her books and journals thus developing an interest in medicine. When his family physician learned of his interest, he insisted that he do his pre-med studies at Haverford College. Berlin is not sure why, because the physician had not gone there, nor had any of his children.

Berlin graduated from Haverford (1958) with a B.A. with honors and was elected to Phi Beta Kappa (1958). He majored in chemistry with special interests in synthetic organic chemistry and physical chemistry. One of his great experiences at Haverford was the Phillips Visitors Program which was organized to bring distinguished visitors to the campus to meet with small student groups. Berlin was chosen to host Nobel Laureate Linus Pauling who gave a lecture on how he discovered the alpha helix structure in proteins and the molecular error in sickle cell anemia.

He received his M.D. *cum laude* from Harvard Medical School (1962) with special interests in electrophysiology; pharmacology of methoxamine; and inborn errors of metabolism. He was elected to the Boylston Society at Harvard Medical School(1961).

He completed a Pediatric Internship (1961-62; Dr. Charles Janeway) at the Children's Hospital Medical Center, Boston, MA. He then fulfilled his military service (Berry Plan) as a Senior Assistant Surgeon, USPHS, Laboratory of Biochemical Pharmacology, National Institute of Arthritis and Metabolic Disease, NIH, Bethesda, MD. He was assigned to the laboratory of Dr. Herbert Tabor, one of the legends of biochemistry, and worked with Dr.

Robert T. Schimke, also a legend in biochemistry. He returned to the Children's Hospital Medical Center in Boston for his Pediatric Residency (1965-67; Dr. Charles Janeway).

Berlin began his academic career as an Assistant Professor of Pediatrics at the University of Alabama Medical Center, Birmingham, AL (1967-68; Dr. Herschel Bentley); moving to the George Washington University School of Medicine, Washington, DC as Assistant Professor of Pediatrics (1968-71; Dr. Felix Heald). He concurrently served as Director, Intensive Care Unit, Children's Hospital of the District of Columbia. He was a Markle Scholar in Academic Medicine (1969-74), a competitive and prestigious award to very promising, smart, academic types who were being lost to private practice because they could not afford to stay in academic medicine.

He was appointed to TMSHMC as Associate Professor of Pediatrics in 1971 (as the 2nd faculty appointee in Pediatrics) and Associate Professor of Pharmacology (Dr. Elliot Vesell, Chair) and to Professor of Pediatrics and Professor of Pharmacology in 1975. He concurrently served as Director, Pediatric Inpatient Service (1971-1999), and Director, Pediatric Intensive Care Unit (1971-1980). He had previously (1968) been considered for the Chair of Pediatrics, TMSHMC but declined because he thought that it was premature. Later, when Dr. Nicholas Nelson called him to tell him that he wanted him to move to Hershey, Berlin's response was "I can't do that; last month I purchased and moved into our first home." Nelson's response, in a most sympathetic and supportive fashion, was: "Sell it." Dr. Nicholas Nelson (Chair of Pediatrics) had been Berlin's attending when he was a medical student, an intern, and third year resident; in all, 4 years of interaction. He did come and was promoted/appointed to Professor of Pediatrics (1975-present), and Pharmacology (1975-present); Chief, Division of General Pediatrics (1984-2000); Member, Division of Clinical Pharmacology/Department of Medicine (1978-present); Director, PKU Clinic, and in 1986 was named the University Professor of Pediatrics. A sabbatical year (1979-80) was spent at the Children's

Hospital of Philadelphia in the laboratory of Dr. Sumner Yaffe studying the excretion of drugs in human milk.

In addition to his clinical and research activities, he served as Assistant Dean for Student Affairs (1972-87) and Chairman, Medical Student Selection Committee (1972-1975 and 1985-86). In this position he was responsible for all of student affairs including admissions, financial aid, academic progress, and preparing the Dean's letter for residency applications of the 4th year medical students. When Waldhausen, Interim Dean, told the Executive Committee (department chairs) that he really needed an Assistant Dean for Student Affairs, Nelson spoke up and said that he was trying to recruit someone who would be perfect for that job. The person was Berlin.

Berlin has received numerous awards for his teaching and research. He was appointed as an endowed University Professor of Pediatrics in 1986. In 2006, he received the Sumner J. Yaffe Lifetime Achievement Award in Pediatric Pharmacology and Therapeutics, In 2008, He received the Penn State Alumni Association Honorary Award and the Student Pediatric Society endowed the Berlin Leadership and Service Award; and the new Penn State Children's Hospital library is named the Cheston M. Berlin, Jr Library.

Dr. Berlin's clinical and research interests are in the regulation of enzyme levels and activities in tissues, general pediatrics, pediatric pharmacology, neuromuscular diseases, lactation, lupus antibodies, excretion of drugs and chemicals in human milk, phenylketonuria (PKU), and treatment of tic disorders including Tourette syndrome. He continues as the Director of the PKU Clinic at TMSHMC.

DEPARTMENT of PEDIATRICS, DIVISION of PEDIATRIC GENETICS – ROGER LADDA, M.D. was the founding Chief of the Division of Human Genetics, Growth and Development (1973-).

Dr. Ladda was born (10/28/36) Highland, IL, and raised in Lebanon, IL. His father was in the construction business, building houses. He helped his father during the summers, and briefly considered a career in architecture because he liked to draw, and often did designs for his father's clients. However, pouring concrete in the hot Illinois sun convinced him of his life-long desire to be a physician. He excelled in science and was encouraged by one of his teachers. Under her supervision, he did a lot of science projects. In his sophomore year, he started doing electron microscopy at the Washington University in St. Louis, MO. As a result, he won the top award in the St. Louis Science Fair in 1955. The top prize was a full ride to Wesleyan for undergraduate study.

His early exposure to medicine was through his family physician. He worked with another family physician during the summers, and often gave hormone and vitamin injections to older women.

He graduated from Wesleyan ('58, A.B., Honors) after three years and applied to Washington University, University of Chicago, and the University of Illinois for medical school. He chose the University of Chicago. As a result of his experience in electron microscopy, he worked in a research laboratory in hematology/oncology. They had a major research program studying erythrocytes. He was chosen to work in the laboratory of Marcel Bessis (1960-61, Fullbright Scholar) in Paris, France who was considered to be one of the leaders in the study of ultrastructure of blood cells. After his one year he returned to the University of Chicago to complete his M.D. (1963). From his laboratory research, he strongly considered a career in pathology, and doing a Ph.D. After graduation, he elected to stay at the University of Chicago to do a pathology fellowship (1963-64). However, after his 60th autopsy secondary to a myocardial infarction, he decided that pathology was not for him.

He was leaning towards a career in Pediatrics when he was working with an adult nephrologist, John Arnold, who had collaborated with Dr. Alf Alving, an early malaria investigator. Dr. Arnold had received a large malaria grant from the Department of Defense to study malaria infections at the University of Missouri, Kansas City, MO. He was looking for someone to study the cell cycle of the malaria parasite, especially differentiation-dedifferentiation, so Ladda went there (1965) thinking he would then do a residency at either the University of Kansas or the University of Missouri, but neither materialized. Although he found that to be a superb learning experience, he realized that without having completed a residency, his career was at a stand-still.

Ladda then went to the University of Washington Children's Hospital in Seattle, WA. After his first year of pediatric residency, and facing the draft, he signed up to join the Army (Berry Plan). He was assigned to the Walter Reed Army Institute for Research (WRAIR) in Washington, D.C. ((1967-70), where he also collaborated with investigators at Georgetown University and the NIH.

After his discharge from the military, he was a Junior Assistant Resident at the Children's Hospital Medical Center, Boston, MA (1970-71), followed by being Assistant Resident (1971-72) in Medicine at Harvard. He continued as Clinical and Research Fellow at the Massachusetts General Hospital, Harvard (1972-74).

In 1973, he was contacted by Dr. Nelson about a faculty position in the Department of Pediatrics. On his first visit, he was impressed with the "first generation" of faculty (Nelson, Berlin, Maisels, and Kulin). There was an atmosphere of warmth, concern, and expectations; and there were no limitations. All of this was an excellent fit with his goal of working in an atmosphere where he had an opportunity to be independent, creative, and if they succeeded, they succeeded because of their own efforts; if they did not, it would be their own fault. In sum, a grand opportunity to continue the experiment.

Upon his arrival, he established a cytogenetics laboratory. There had been a small chromosomal laboratory in Pathology. He was given free rein to incorporate that into his new cytogenetics laboratory in Pediatrics. He also continued as a clinician and ward attending and developed his research program which had evolved into a study of growth factors.

He credits part of his success to the collegial support of several individuals; Wayne Bardin (Medicine, Endocrinology), Elliot Vesell (Pharmacology), Bryce Munger (Anatomy), C. Max Lang (Comparative Medicine), Al Vastyan (Humanities), Richard Naeye (Pathology), Chet Berlin and Jeff Maisels (Pediatrics), etc. It was very collegial and oriented towards the centrality of the institution, as opposed to individual efforts.

DEPARTMENT of PEDIATRICS, Division of INFECTIOUS DISEASES – JOHN DOSSETT, M.D.

Dr. Dossett was born in Mobile, AL on July 21, 1938 and was raised in the farming area of Southern and Central MS. He states his family was a poor "blue collar" farming family, and he was the first in his family to attend college. Growing up, skills in cotton picking were more highly valued than athletic prowess or academic accomplishments. In high school, he always had a part-time job which allowed him to buy his clothes and have some spending money. When he finished high school, his family was living in Clinton, MS, the home of Mississippi College where he attended and received his bachelor's degree in 1960. He received his M.D. degree from the University of Alabama in 1964. He financed his undergraduate and medical education by holding part-time jobs, and after 1959, with student loans. Medical school was followed by three years of Pediatric Residency and a two year fellowship in infectious diseases in the Department of Pediatrics at the University of Minnesota. During his two year fellowship, he worked in the laboratory of Dr. Paul Quie, a renowned investigator in the field. This was a very productive research experience for Dr. Dossett. He was the author or coauthor of 7 publications resulting from his work with Dr. Quie and three presentations at national meetings. At the end of his fellowship, he fulfilled his Berry Plan military obligation serving as a Major in the USAF at Andrews Air Force Base in Washington, D.C.

Near the completion of his military service, Dr. Dossett was considering his future and favoring an academic career. He had offers from a number of University Pediatric Departments including TMSHMC. He made the decision to accept the Hershey position because of the semi-rural setting of the area, the excitement and challenges of starting a new medical school, and his respect and admiration for the founding Chairman of Pediatrics (Dr. Nicholas Nelson). Dr. Dossett was one of the first three faculty recruits when the department opened in July, 1971. He was appointed as Assistant Professor and Chief of Pediatric Infectious Diseases in 1971. He was promoted to Associate Professor in 1977 and to Professor in 1993.

From 1971 to 1976, Dr. Dossett was the only Infectious Disease Specialist on the staff of the Medical Center, providing consultation services to all clinical departments. In 1976, Dr. Robert Aber, an Infectious Disease Specialist joined the Department of Medicine. The Infectious Disease Program continued as a joint Medicine-Pediatric Program until 1989 when the program split into separate divisions in each department. Dr. Dossett continued as Chief of Pediatric Infectious Diseases until 2009.

Although Dr. Dossett had been a very productive laboratory based investigator during his fellowship, he did not establish such a program in Hershey. He focused his professional activities on patient care and education. In addition he served on many medical center and university committees, including two terms as president of the Faculty Organization. He feels that the contribution he values most was his work on the Biomedical Ethics Committee. In 1986, he was the founding chair of that committee and served for 20 years, 14 as chair.

DEPARTMENT of PEDIATRICS, DIVISION of PEDIATRIC NEONATOLOGY – M. JEFFREY MAISELS, M.B.,B.Ch., D.Sc. (Med); founding Chief (1972-86).

Maisels was born in Johannesburg, South Africa on October 18, 1937. His father was a well-known lawyer, and perhaps best known for his defense of Nelson Mandela and others in the famous South African Treason Trial (1959-61). His mother also had a strong influence on his life. She was a homemaker in the tradition of those days but was very involved in community events and community services.

His grandparents came from Eastern Europe. His paternal grandparents came from Lithuania in 1893, and his maternal grandparents from Poland in 1895; both because of a combination of the economic conditions in Europe and the anti-Jewish discrimination and pogroms.

He chose medicine almost by a process of elimination. His uncle was involved in business, but Maisels had no idea what business people did. He couldn't be an architect because he couldn't draw. He was poor at math, so that eliminated engineering. His decision really came down to law or medicine; and he decided on medicine. He did have a great-uncle whom was the first chief of Urology at the Johannesburg General Hospital. Also, he had a very good role model in the family's GP (General Practitioner). It was the custom at that time to make house calls in the morning and have office visits in the afternoon. Maisels had never been in a doctor's office until he left South Africa.

Maisels went to the University of Witwatersrand in Johannesburg and received his M.B., B.Ch. (Bachelor of Medicine and Bachelor of Surgery) in 1961. The basic science courses were adequate, and they had wonderful clinicians who taught at the bedside with rounds in the classic Socratic manner of teaching. It was a common practice for the faculty to humiliate the students; in fact, if you weren't humiliated at least once a day, you felt as though you were being ignored.

A first year internship was required, which was six months of medicine and six months of surgery (1962). He knew that he was not going to be a surgeon so, following his internship, he went into his pediatric residency at the Baragwanath Hospital which was probably the largest hospital in the Southern Hemisphere. This was during the apartheid era and it was an all-black hospital with 2,000 beds, but at any given time usually had about 3,000 patients; the remaining patients were sleeping two to a bed, on the floor or in a chair. There were 250 pediatric beds divided into four wards, and a premature nursery with 150 beds. In those days they did not ventilate any babies; it was survival of the fittest. It was an incredible experience because there was a tremendous amount of pathology. In outpatient clinic, an average of 70 patients a day appeared; mostly acute illnesses. On night call there were two residents covering about 250 beds and about 150 premature babies. He did 3 years of pediatric training there (1962-65).

His medical training took place during the height of the apartheid era in South Africa and he decided he would leave South Africa when he finished his training. He considered different opportunities and decided he would come to the United States to complete some training, and perhaps subspecialty training. He wanted to do what other pediatricians were doing in South Africa, i.e., act as a pediatric consultant. GPs took care of children. If they had a problem, they referred them to a pediatric specialist.

During the South African Treason Trial, his father became a friend of Prof. Erwin Griswold, Dean of Harvard Law School, who had been at the trial as an observer. Maisels' father wrote Griswold asking if he would help his son get a residency program around the Boston area. He arrived in Boston in January, 1966 and spent a year at the North Shore Children's Hospital in Salem, MA. At the end of the year, Dr. Janeway asked him to be the Chief Resident in the outpatient department at Boston Children's Hospital. After six months, Maisels decided that he was interested in neonatology and applied to the program at Boston Lying-in Hospital (now Brigham and Womens). Dr. Clement Smith was the head of the program, and had been Dr. Nick Nelson's mentor (founding chair of pediatrics at TMSHMC).

He soon learned that the fellowship was a research fellowship. Maisels had absolutely no idea what research was about. Nick Nelson (later the founding Chair of Pediatrics at TMSHMC) had him review some research papers describing a technique for measuring carbon monoxide production, a direct measurement of heme catabolism, and bilirubin production. He adapted the technique to newborn infants and his first paper on carbon monoxide in newborns was published in 1971 in the *Journal of Clinical Investigation*.

He had completed 18 months of his neonatal fellowship when he was drafted into the U.S. Army. He tried to get into the USPHS (NIH) but did not qualify since he was a foreigner. Dr. David Nathan (then chief of hematology at the Boston's Children's Hospital) called a colleague of his at the Walter Reed Army Institute for Research (WRAIR), Dr. Marcel Conrad, and told him of Maisels' training and experience. Conrad agreed to have him assigned to the WRAIR but he would have to serve three years instead of the usual two. He achieved the rank of Lt. Colonel.

As he was finishing his military service (1971), Dr. Nick Nelson asked him to come for an interview. He was impressed with the facility and the faculty, and agreed to come to Hershey. He was appointed as an Assistant Professor of Pediatrics and Obstetrics and Gynecology in 1972, promoted to Associate Professor in 1975, and to Professor in 1980.

When Maisels arrived, the neonatal intensive care unit was not yet built. His vision was to build a neonatal unit from scratch. He did so with limited faculty resources. He was on call every night for the first three years. Finally, he was able to recruit Dr. Keith Marks, first as a Fellow, then as a faculty member. They developed a research program, and he continued his research with jaundiced babies. They were now on the cutting edge of neonatology and they proceeded to regionalize South Central Pennsylvania. At one stage, they were getting babies referred to them from 60 hospitals in 24 Pennsylvania counties.

He was a member of 20 organizations and served on the editorial boards of Pediatrics and as chair of the Sub Board of Neonatal-Perinatal Medicine of the American Board of Pediatrics The focus of his research was jaundice and hyperbilirubinemia, but he has also widely published in other areas of neonatology. He has written over 200 peer-reviewed and invited publications and book chapters and 2 books on jaundice in the newborn.

He left TMSHMC to be the Physician-in-Chief at the Beaumont Children's Hospital, and subsequently, Professor and Founding Chair, Department of Pediatrics, Oakland University William Beaumont School of Medicine, Royal Oak, MI. He thoroughly enjoyed his time at TMSHMC, especially clinical and research activities, but was beginning to feel "burnt out" by teaching. i.e. he found himself repeating the same information over and over to rotating medical students and residents. Still, there was nothing making him leave Hershey, except that he was looking for the opportunity to be a chair.

In 2007 he received the Richardson Award from the Society for Pediatric Research for lifetime contributions to pediatric research and, in the same year, he received the Virginia Apgar award, which he described as a sort of Hall of Fame of neonatologists. It is the American Academy of Pediatrics, Neonatal-Perinatal Section award and is given annually to one individual, from anywhere in the world, in recognition of outstanding contributions to perinatal medicine.

He received the D.Sc. in 2008 for a thesis submitted to his medical school in Johannesburg that was based on 40 years of research in jaundiced newborns.

He was interviewed for the Chair of Pediatrics at Hershey. He was very interested in the position but had mixed feelings about leaving Beaumont as he had only been there for one year and was actively engaged in recruiting.

DEPARTMENT of PEDIATRICS, PEDIATRIC NEPHROLOGY -- STEVEN J. WASSNER, M.D., FAAP; founding Chief of Pediatric Nephrology (1978-).

Dr. Wassner was born December 16, 1946 in New York, NY. His parents were both immigrants to this country; his mother in 1920, and his father in 1939. His mother was a seamstress and worked for the International Ladies Garment Workers union. His father was an interpreter and translator for the Federal Government Immigration and Naturalization Service. He has an older sister who has a Ph.D. in Psychology, and works as a psychologist in CA.

He chose the City College of New York for his undergraduate degree (B.S., 1968), and went to New York University for medical school M.D. (1972). He was very impressed with his pediatrics rotation and decided to make that his career choice. He interned at the Children's Hospital of Los Angeles because "everyone was going to California" at that time. He did his residency and a Fellowship in Pediatric Nephrology at the same institution. His original plan was to be a "West coaster" for three years, then return to New York as a general pediatrician and open a practice in Long Island which for a New York City boy was sort of like dying and going to Heaven. However, during his internship and residency, he quickly realized that he was not suited to be an outpatient pediatrician, but rather to be on the inpatient service, particularly in endocrinology and nephrology.

He had an interest in research. The head of nephrology (Ellen Lieberman) at LA Children's told him that they did not really have much of a research program there. She had just returned from a sabbatical at UC San Francisco and suggested that Wassner do a fellowship there, which probably had the most distinguished nephrology program in the world.

After completing his training, he began to look for a job, but there were not many openings. He saw an advertisement in a non-descript journal indicating a position at Hershey. He wrote a letter to Nelson (founding chair of Pediatrics), and was invited for an interview. Nelson later told him the reason he hired him was quite simple; he had money for a hematologist but could not find one, so he hired Wassner.

Wassner told Nelson that his vision was very simple; "I think I can be a good clinician, but I want to come here and do research and teach and you will have to take a chance on me." Nelson agreed to take the chance. Wassner arrived in July, 1978 and immediately started writing two grants; an RO1 to the NIH and one to the Muscular Dystrophy Association; both were funded. He developed an active research program, and was a busy clinician. He did a sabbatical (1985-86) as a Visiting Professor of Human Biochemistry, The Hebrew University, Hadassah Hospital in Jerusalem, Israel. After his sabbatical, he realized that he was more interested in clinical activities and teaching rather than writing grants and doing research. So, he started a pediatric diabetes service and, as the sole physician, built it up to 300 families.

The new chair of Pediatrics (Dr. Ronald Poland) asked him to take over the pediatric residency program. Later, he was asked to serve as vice chair of the department.

DEPARTMENT of PSYCHIATRY -- ANTHONY KALES, M.D., D.H.C. (honorary) founding Chair, 1971-98. Kales was born in Detroit, Mi. His parents had emigrated from Northern Epiros, which is now under Albanian control. He grew up in a very ethnic

Greek home, surrounded by numerous relatives and with strong Greek ties and loyalties.

He graduated from Wayne State University in 1956 with High Distinction and as a member of Phi Beta Kappa Honor Society. After graduation from Wayne State University School of Medicine in 1959 (3 years), he went to UCLA, completing his psychiatry residency in 1963. He remained on the faculty at UCLA, attaining the rank of Professor in 1971.

Kales was appointed Professor and Chairman of the Department of Psychiatry, TMSHMC in 1971. From 1984-2001 he was also the Director of the Central Pennsylvania Psychiatric Institute which is one of three state-funded training and research institutes for the Commonwealth of PA Psychiatric Care. This had to be a difficult task, albeit a very worthy one, because he dealt directly with a member of the Pennsylvania Legislature, rather than go through the University who he thought might compromise the University's appropriation.

Kales' most notable accomplishments include co-authoring a sleep stage scoring manual in 1968 which remains the fundamental criterion to evaluate the effectiveness of hypnotics and psychoactive drugs. He has made many contributions to the understanding of sleep and its various disorders, including insomnia, sleepwalking, night terrors, bedwetting, sleep apnea, and narcolepsy. He has published over 300 articles and six books. He has received many awards and honors including membership in Phi Beta Kappa and Alpha Omega Alpha, the highest undergraduate university and medical student awards, and Honorary Doctorate Degree (*Doctor Honoris Causa*) from the University of Athens School of Medicine, Greece.

Kales built a strong academic Department of Psychiatry, focusing on education, research, and patient care. He had developed a manual, outlining the steps to develop a diagnosis and treatment of psychiatric illness which was an important asset in his education activities. His sleep research program is recognized internationally.

DEPARTMENT of RADIOLOGY -- WILLIAM WEIDNER, M., founding Chair, 1971-87. Weidner was born November 30, 1928 in Milwaukee, WI. He graduated from Milton Union High School in 1945, then attended Milton College (1945-47) both in Milton, WI. He transferred to the University of Wisconsin, Madison, WI, receiving his B.S. in 1949, and M.D. degree in 1952 (3 years). He did a rotating internship (1952-53) at the Medical College of Virginia Hospitals, Richmond, VA. From 1953-56, he served as Lt, MC, USNR (Flight Surgeon). After his military service (Berry Plan), he completed a residency in General Surgery (1956-57), University of Washington VA Hospital, Seattle, WA; and a residency in radiology (1958-61), LAC-USC Medical Center, Los Angeles, CA. From 1961-63, he worked at the Huntington Memorial Hospital, Pasadena, CA. He was a NIH Fellow in neuroradiology, University of California for Health Sciences, Los Angeles, CA. He then had a series of appointments:

1964-68 Associate Professor of Radiology, UCLA Center for the Health Sciences, and 1965-68 Chief Radiologist, Harbor General Hospital, Torrance, CA 1968-69 Professor of Radiology, Chairman, Diagnostic Radiology, Medical College of Virginia Hospital, Richmond, VA 1969-71 Professor of Radiology, University of Oklahoma Hospitals, Oklahoma City, OK

Weidner was appointed Professor and Chair, TMSHMC in 1971. He concurrently served as Associate Dean for Patient Care (1974-78). He stepped down as Chair of the Department of Radiology in 1987, but continued to serve as Professor of Radiology and Director of Neuroradiology, Angiography and Interventional Radiology (1987-89).

Weidner was an excellent radiologist, a consummate angiographer and neuroradiologist; and received several research grants. He has a long list of special awards, honors, and appointments (32) and membership in 24 professional organizations. He presented 98 scientific papers/exhibits at local, regional, national, and international meetings. Weidner is the author/co-author of 76 scientific publications and 1 book. He received a Letter of Commendation from the

Governor of Pennsylvania for his "dedication and leadership in the field of Radiology and to the Hershey Medical Center".

The Department of Radiology was originally designed in a vertical mode by location, then gradually changed to a horizontal mode. However, with electronic technology, the imaging equipment is now being dispersed to the areas of patient care.

DEPARTMENTS of RADIOLOGY and MEDICINE -- G. VICTOR ROHRER, M.D., 1973-98.

Rohrer was born November 8, 1933 in Ashland, KS. He was raised on a ranch near the Kansas-Oklahoma border.

Rohrer received his B.S. from the Oklahoma State University, Stillwater, OK (1954), and M.D. degree from The University of Oklahoma School of Medicine, Oklahoma City, OK (1958). He did his internship at the Cincinnati General Hospital, Cincinnati, OH, then returned to the University of Oklahoma as an Internal Medicine Resident (1959-61), Gastroenterology Trainee/NIAMS (1961-62), Gastroenterology Special Research Fellow/NIAMS (1962-63), Medicine Chief Resident (1963-64), and Diagnostic Radiology Resident (1964-69).

Rohrer began his academic career at the University of Oklahoma as Assistant Professor of Medicine (1964-69), Assistant Professor of Radiology (1966-69). He was promoted to Associate Professor of Medicine and Radiology (1969-71). He worked with Weidner at the University of Oklahoma, who recruited him to TMSHMC in 1971 as Associate Professor of Radiology and Medicine. He was named Vice Chair of the department in 1972, and promoted to Professor of Radiology and Medicine in 1973. He concurrently served as Director, Diagnostic Radiology Residency Program (1977-82), Associate Dean for Patient Care (1982-86), and Associate Dean for Clinical Affairs (1987-1993). He gave up his administrative appointments in 1993, and remained as a Professor of Radiology doing clinical radiology and working with residents until his retirement in 1998. He served on 50 committees at TMSHMC.

He is the author/co-author of 24 scientific publications. He is the recipient of the Gold Medallion Award from the Pennsylvania Radiological Society for outstanding contributions (2001), and the G. Victor Rohrer Professorship in Radiological Education that was established in his honor by former residents (2004).

DEPARTMENT of RADIOLOGY, DIVISION OF HEALTH PHYSICS -- KENNETH L. MILLER, B.S., M.S., founding Chief, 1971-2008.

Miller was born August 14, 1943 in Plum Run Hollow (Lock Haven), PA. His father completed the 6th or 7th grade, his mother the 3rd grade. His mother came from a hard-scrapple farm where cheap labor was more important than education. His father worked as a laborer hauling coal and ice until he got a job as a welder for Piper Aircraft. Although his mother had little formal education, she taught him to read before he started the first grade. He went to a one room school, with one teacher and 8 grades. He excelled in school, and often took reading and math classes with students who were one or two grades ahead of him. He had a love of reading and an insatiable desire for learning.

Miller graduated from high school with 1500 SAT scores and a Piper Aircraft Scholarship that paid $300/year. He applied to college and, after graduation from high school, married his high school sweet heart. Although he was accepted by all of the schools to which he applied, he chose Lock Haven State College because it was the only one he could afford. In college, he acquired a triple major in mathematics, physics, and general science (in 3 years) and worked part time at 3 jobs, 40-60 hours/week. His advisor recommended that he take the requisite teaching courses and do student teaching.

He received his B.S. in 1965, and accepted a teaching position in the Port Allegheny School System, PA. He thoroughly enjoyed teaching but, to obtain permanent certification as a teacher, he would have to acquire 24 additional credits beyond the bachelor's degree. He decided to leave teaching and find a job that paid more so he could go back to school. He was hired by Piper Aircraft to be an aeronautical engineer. Since he had never had a course in drafting, he was placed in the drafting department for 6 months. During that time, the aircraft industry took a nose dive. They told him that he would have to wait for the economy to improve, and receive the salary level that was promised.

He accepted a position at TPSU in 1966 as Health Physics Assistant, and permission to take courses at a 75% discount. During the next 3 years, he accumulated 24 credits in computer science, nuclear physics, nuclear engineering, and biophysics.

In 1969, he took a leave of absence from TPSU to accept a PHS Fellowship at the University of Pittsburgh. After 12 months at the University of Pittsburgh, he completed 64 graduate credits, completed a research project and thesis defense; receiving the M.S. degree in 1970.

Miller returned to TPSU but things did not work out as planned. He decided to find a position where he could run his own show. He was offered positions at Rutgers University, National Accelerator Laboratory, and the nuclear Navy. He had also been contacted by TMSHMC. Dr Harrell was concerned with the oversight of the Hershey Program from TPSU 90 miles away and, if the Medical Center were to be in control of its' own destiny, it would need to develop its own radiation safety programs, obtain its own licenses, and run its own show. Miller accepted the challenge and was given free rein to do whatever was necessary to accomplish these objectives.

Miller's goal was to develop one of the best, if not the best, radiation safety program in the country. He did this by first developing an excellent radiation safety manual that was sufficiently inclusive yet short enough for anyone to read and clear enough for everyone to understand. He developed many techniques and equipment to safely work with radioactive materials. An important aspect of the success of his program was his attitude that he was not a police officer and policing was not his responsibility; he was insistent, but he was also fair and reasonable.

Miller was a forerunner in a number of innovations, e.g. trash compaction of radioactive waste, a system to use waste liquid scintillation fluids as supplementary fuel in the animal crematorium, radioactive xenon trapping system, etc.

Shortly after his arrival at TMSHMC, and long before the nuclear incident, Miller was contacted by the Three Mile Island Power Plant (TMI) and asked to develop a medical radiation emergency plan for the plant. This resulted in a formal agreement between the medical center and the owners of TMI. As a part of this agreement, TMSHMC agreed to accept and provide care, treatment and decontamination for any radiation accident victims from TMI. In return, TMI agreed to help with the annual training of the Emergency Department (ED) staff, provide supplies and equipment for use with radiation accident victims and cover the costs of decontamination of rooms and equipment or replacement of equipment that could not be decontaminated.

When the accident occurred at TMI on March 28, 1979, TMSHMC and Miller had the spotlight focused on them. Miller believes that the most significant thing that he did during the accident was to interpret what was going on and put it into words that everyone could understand.

When TMSHMC was asked by the Governor's office to remain open, but transporting all but the seriously ill to other hospitals (costing TMSHMC a loss of approximately $1 million per week) and provide decontamination of people who were caught in a fallout situation, Miller developed a radiation emergency triage program in the Receiving Area of TMSHMC. This simple procedure became the model for the country, and was resurrected and copied extensively after 9/11. Shortly after TMI, the EPA Environmental Monitoring Laboratory was established in Middletown, PA. Eight years later, the EPA could not figure out how they could gracefully back out of the environmental monitoring business. Miller submitted a proposal to transfer the laboratory to TMSHMC, fully funded, first by the EPA, then by the Bureau of Radiation Protection. Although it was eventually closed, it did bring some sophisticated analytical counting equipment to the Health Physics Group and several hundred thousand dollars a year for operation of the laboratory.

Miller received the Elda E. Anderson Award from the Health Physics Society; the highest recognition given to a Health Physicist who has had significant success prior to the age of 40. This award typically denotes those who will become significant contributors to the Society and the profession in the future.

Miller has published 122 scientific publications, 24 editorials, 55 internet publications, 17 books, and 7 booklets. Nearly everything he published was of practical health physics nature and designed to help others. He is especially proud of the accomplishments he made as Editor-in-Chief of the *Health Physics Journal*. He also developed a new scientific journal, *Operational Radiation Safety*.

Upon his retirement from TMSHMC as Emeritus Professor of Radiology, the Department of Radiology endowed the Chair of Radiology in his name.

DEPARTMENT of SURGERY -- JOHN A. WALDHAUSEN, M.D. founding Chair, 1969-94. He was born May 22, 1929, in NY, NY (died May 15, 2012); he was an American-born US citizen who had spent seven years of his youth in the middle of World War II in Nazi, Germany. He has published his autobiography: *Finding Home in a World at War, 1929-1963*, John A. Waldhausen, 2005, Gateway Press, Inc, Baltimore, MD, www.gatewaypress.com.

His parents were born and raised in Germany. His father was employed by Siemens Corporation, and when he announced that he was being promoted to Siemens Corporation, North America, his family quickly arranged for his marriage, and they sailed to the US.

When World War II broke out with the invasion of Poland by Germany, his parents believed that it was going to be a long war, perhaps 5 years; it would be a disastrous war, involving the entire world; and Germany would ultimately lose because of the huge manufacturing capacity of the U.S. Although neither of his parents were very much involved with Adolf Hitler and the Nazis, his family, as a whole, had a long history of serving Germany either in the Army or government. Thus, they felt more German than American. His father believed that he would be seen as an enemy-and would be either in Germany or the US-and they might be put in a camp, similar to the Japanese. They decided to return to Germany.

His life and education were disrupted by the war. At the end of the war, since he was a U. S. citizen, the authorities decided that he should return to the U.S. on a troop transport ship. He went to NYC and lived with a former employee of his fathers at Siemens. He applied to Columbia and several other colleges, but they all said no. While in Germany, he had met an Army Chaplain who was now a parish priest and had said to look him up if he ever needed help. He wrote him a letter but did not receive a reply. One night, he received a telephone call from the priest who was now head of a small college in Great Falls, Montana; 300 students, but accredited. He was given a full scholarship but had to have a job for living expenses. He got a job in a restaurant doing menial tasks. However he lost that job when he had a skiing accident. He then got a job in a local hospital as an orderly. He was asked if he would like to work in the lab and, when he learned the procedures, take night call. Then he was offered the opportunity to work for a surgical pathologist.

He graduated from the University of Great Falls, Great Falls, MT with a B.S. *cum laude* (Chemistry) in 1950 (after 3 years of undergraduate education). He applied to 8 medical schools, mainly in the East and was accepted by 4 schools. He accepted the offer from the St. Louis University School of Medicine in 1950, and received his M.D. degree in 1954. He was elected to the Alpha Omega Alpha Honor Medical Society (1953), and received the C.V. Mosby award for Outstanding Scholarship in Medicine (1954). He was the best student in medicine but he thought he could combine medicine and surgery and chose the latter. He interned in Surgery (1954-55) at The Johns Hopkins Hospital, Baltimore, MD. He remained at Hopkins for a Research Fellowship in Surgery (1955-56), then as an Assistant Resident and Assistant Instructor in Surgery (1956-57). He served two years in the U.S. Public Health Service, Clinic of Surgery, NHLBI/NIH, Bethesda, MD (1957-59). He was Assistant Resident, Surgery, Hospital of the University of Pennsylvania, Philadelphia, PA (1959). He then was the Chief Resident in Surgery, Indiana University Medical Center, Indianapolis, IN (1960-62).

His goal was ultimately to run his own department of surgery, with the youthful view that such would clearly be better than those led by many of the then current surgery chairmen. Although the initial faculty size for the Department of Surgery was 8, he envisioned a minimum of 30, covering all of the surgical subspecialties, all providing clinical excellence and very productive in research. He was committed to his faculty and department but was always collegial to his colleagues in other departments. Perhaps his greatest attribute was that he led by example.

Waldhausen began his academic career at the Indiana University School of Medicine, Indianapolis, IN as an Instructor in Surgery (1961-63), and promoted to Assistant Professor (1963-66). He was appointed Associate Professor in Surgery at the University of Pennsylvania, Philadelphia, PA (1966-70), and concurrently as Associate Director of the Cardiovascular Research Institute (1967-70).

He was recruited to TMSHMC in 1969 as Professor and Chairman of the Department of Surgery (although the first year he worked 4 days at Penn and 3 days at Hershey each week). He served, concurrently, as Interim Vice President for Health Affairs and Dean (1972-73); and Associate Dean for Health Care (1973-75); Director, Section of Surgical Sciences, and Surgeon-in-Chief, University Hospital (1993-94) and Executive Director, University Physicians (1994-96). He was named the John W. Oswald Professor of Surgery in 1983.

Waldhausen was a member of 29 medical organizations and held multiple offices in 16 professional associations. He has received numerous awards and honors. He has served on 7 editorial boards, 26 committees, and 59 invited professorships and lectures.

His research interests include surgery of congenital and acquired heart disease and circulatory changes associated with cardiovascular surgery. He is the author/co-author of 231 manuscripts in peer-reviewed journals, and 46 books and book chapters.

Walhausen recruited the best and the brightest. He consistently pushed his faculty, in a positive manner, to excel in surgical expertise and compassionate patient care. As a young chair, his faculty were also young and he paid particular attention to their growth and development including their participation in their professional organizations.

DEPARTMENT of SURGERY, CARDIOVASCULAR and ARTIFICIAL ORGANS -- WILLIAM S(huler) PIERCE, M.D., D.Sc. (honorary) was born January 12, 1937 in Wilkes-Barre, PA. He went to high school at the Wyoming Seminary, Kingston, PA and graduated *cum laude* in 1954. He entered Lehigh University, Bethlehem, PA, graduating with a B.S. in Chemical Engineering with Highest Honors in 1958. He also received the Diefenderfer Award—Qualitative Analysis Award (1956), Chandler Award for the highest grades in Chemical and Chemical Engineering (1956-58), Pi Mu Epsilon Mathematics Honorary Society (1956), and Tau Beta Pi Engineering Honorary Society (1956). He has subsequently been the recipient of 18 different awards.

He received his M.D. degree from the University of Pennsylvania School of Medicine, Philadelphia, PA in 1962. He was elected to Alpha Omega Alpha (medical honorary society) in 1962. He was a Rotating Intern at the Hospital of the University of Pennsylvania (1962-63) and Assistant Resident in Surgery (1963-65). He fulfilled his military obligation (Berry Plan) by serving as a Lieutenant Commander, Surgeon, USPHS, Clinical Associate, Surgical Section, National Heart Institute, NIH (1965-67). He then returned to the Hospital of the University of Pennsylvania as Assistant Resident in Surgery (1967-68), Resident in Surgery (1968-69), and Chief Resident in Surgery (1969-70).

Pierce began his academic career at TMSHMC as an Assistant Professor in 1970, promoted to Associate Professor in 1973, and Professor in 1977. He concurrently served as Chief, Division of Artificial Organs (1983-91); appointed as the Jane A. Fetter Professor of Surgery (1986-97) and the Evan Pugh Professor of Surgery in 1986; Chief, Division of Cardiothoracic Surgery (1991-95); Director of Research and Vice Chair, Department of Surgery (1995-97).

He is a member of 28 professional societies, served on 34 University committees, 24 national committees, and 5 international committees. He has served on 11 editorial boards; and received multiple patents. He is the author/co-author of 285 publications in peer-reviewed journals; 91 book chapters, and 2 books. Pierce has served as Visiting Professor at 48 institutions, and has given 139 invited presentations.

He is internationally known for his development of the left heart assist device, and the artificial heart.

DEPARTMENT of SURGERY, DIVISION of GENERAL SURGERY -- DAVID L. NAHRWOLD, M.D., founding Chief (1974-82). He was born December 21, 1936 in Fort Wayne, IN. His father was a physician and he relied heavily on him for career advice. He attended Washington University, St Louis, MO for one year (1953-54). He was an average student, and not impressed with the faculty. Since his career goal was to pursue a career in medicine, his father suggested that he talk to the Dean at the Indiana University School of Medicine. He did so, on Easter Sunday, while he was home for spring break. The dean told him that since he was not performing to his potential at Washington University, was a resident of IN, why not transfer to the Indiana University. He did so, and received an A.B. from Indiana University, Bloomington, IN (1954-56).

After 3 years of undergraduate education, he attended Indiana University School of Medicine, Indianapolis, IN (1956-60) where he received his M.D. degree. He was elected to the Alpha Omega Alpha.

Nahrwold completed his internship in straight surgery (1960-61) at Indiana University Medical Center, Indianapolis, IN and residency in general and thoracic surgery (1961-65) at the same institution. While there, he became good friends with Dr. John Waldhausen who would later become Chair of Surgery at TMSHMC. They had many discussions on the ideal department of surgery at an academic medical center; albeit much of which was based on what not to do. He was a Postdoctoral Scholar in Gastrointestinal Surgery, University of California at Los Angeles (1965-66).

As a result of the military draft (Berry Plan), he served as General and Thoracic Surgeon, US Army, South Vietnam (1966-67). He found this assignment to be relatively unproductive; he was at a field hospital with a light patient load. Fortunately, they had a well-stocked library and he spent a lot of time reading. He was then transferred to the General Leonard Wood Hospital, MO (1967-68) and served as Chief of General Surgery (1968).

Nahrwold began his academic career as an Assistant Professor of Surgery at Indiana University School of Medicine (1968-70). He was recruited to TMSHMC by Waldhausen as an Associate Professor of Surgery (1970-73), and promoted to Professor (1973-82). He concurrently served as Chief, Division of General Surgery (1974-82), Vice-Chairman, Department of Surgery (1971-82), Associate Dean for Patient Care (Chief of Staff) (1978-80), and Associate Provost and Dean for Health Affairs (1980-82). He was recruited by Northwestern University Medical School as the Loyal and Edith Davis Professor and Chairman, Department of Surgery (1982-97); and Surgeon-in-Chief, Northwestern Memorial Hospital (1982-97). He remained as Professor of Surgery and Executive Associate Dean for Clinical Affairs (1997-99). After retiring from Northwestern, he served as Interim Director of the American College of Surgeons (1999-2000).

Nahrwold established a productive research program, publishing 213 manuscripts in peer-reviewed journals. He was a member of 25 professional societies and organizations. He was an active member of 34 organizations, serving as an officer in many; and served on the editorial board of 12 journals. He is the recipient of many honors and awards, including the David L. Nahrwold Professorship at TMSHMC.

DEPARTMENT of SURGERY, DIVISION of GENERAL SURGERY -- WILLIAM E. DeMUTH, M.D., Jr

was born April 3, 1921. He received a B.S. from Franklin and Marshall College, Lancaster, PA in 1943. He was drafted into the military and on the basis of an aptitude test, was placed in the US Army Specialist Training Program (1943-46). He received his M.D. degree in 1946 (3 years) from the University of Pennsylvania, Philadelphia, PA. He completed his internship (1946-47) at the Hospital of the University of Pennsylvania, and received a Fellowship in the Harrison Department of Surgical Research (1947-48). He then returned to active duty with the US Army, rising from 1st Lt to Captain (1948-50). During that time, he was assigned as Assistant Chief of Orthopedic Surgery, Valley Forge General Hospital (1948-49), and Chief, Surgical Service, 376 Station Hospital, Japan (1949-50).

DeMuth began his academic career at the University of Pennsylvania as an Assistant Instructor in Surgery (1950-52). He was promoted to Instructor (1952-55), and to Associate Professor (1955-67). He also served as:

1955-60 Consultant in Thoracic Surgery, Charles Miner State Hospital Tuberculosis), Hamburg, PA 1960 Consultant, Samuel Dixon State Hospital, Mont Alto, PA 1955-71 Chief of Surgery, Carlisle Hospital, Carlisle, PA 1963-71 Thoracic Surgeon, Holy Spirit Hospital, Camp Hill, PA 1963-71 Associate in Surgery, Graduate School of Medicine, Philadelphia, PA 1964 Chief of Surgery, MEDICO Unit, Kuala Lipis General Hospital, Kuala Lipis, Mayalsia 1967-69 Assistant Professor of Surgery, University of Pennsylvania 1969-71 Research Associate Professor of Clinical Surgery, Univ of PA School of Medicine

DeMuth was recruited to TMSHMC as Professor of Surgery, primarily for Trauma and Thoracic Surgery (1971-83). He concurrently served as Assistant Dean for Continuing Education (1977-83). He was a member of 24 professional societies, holding multiple offices in several of them. He had a sustained interest in research, and was author/co-author of 85 publications in peer-reviewed journals. It is interesting to note that, during the 1960's when he was primarily in private practice, he drove to the University of Pennsylvania almost every Thursday to pursue his research interests. His research orientation reflected Dr. Harrell's vision of faculty: (1) building on the body of knowledge in their specialty; (2) setting an example for students of how science supports the art of medicine; (3) the importance of attention to detail and the ability to critically analyze the data to share new information with others.

He was always very congenial, further enhancing his teaching skills. His research activities demonstrated his inquiring mind to students and colleagues.

DEPARTMENT of SURGERY, DIVISION of
NEUROSURGERY -- ROBERT B(icknell) PAGE, M.D. He was
born November 17, 1937 in Philadelphia. PA. He graduated from
Amherst College, Amherst, MA in 1959 with a B.A. He received his
M.D. degree in 1963 from the College of Physicians and Surgeons,
Columbia, NY, NY.

He interned at the First (Columbia) Surgical Division, Bellevue
Hospital, NY, NY (1963-64) and did his first year of residency at the
same institution (1964-65). Because of the military draft (Berry Plan),
he served as a Lieutenant (Medical Corps) in the US Naval Reserve
(1965-67). After his military duty, he continued his residency at the
Yale-New Haven Medical Center, CT (1967-68); VA Hospital, West
Haven, CT (1969); and finished as Chief Resident and Instructor at
Yale-New Haven Medical Center (1970-71).

Page was recruited to TMSHMC as an Assistant Professor of
Neurosurgery and Anatomy (1971-77). He was promoted to Associate
Professor (1977-83), and Professor (1983-2003). He concurrently
served as Chairman, Neuroscience Program (1985-91), and Interim
Chairman, Department of Anatomy (1987). He served on the thesis
committee of 8 Ph.D. candidates in Anatomy. He was given the
Faculty Scholar Award, The Pennsylvania State University (1985).
Page was elected to Alpha Omega Alpha for academic scholarship.

He developed an active research program studying the blood
flow in the neurohypophysial capillary bed. He received 6 NIH and
1 American Cancer Society grants to support his research. Initially,
he and the founding chief, Dr. Richard Bergland, would do elective
surgery and, in alternate months, work in their laboratory. Bergland
never wanted a residency program in neurosurgery; he believed that
most were poorly trained. His approach was to take individuals post-
residency, give them the training that they should have received, and
learn how to do research.

Dr. Page is the author/co-author of 52 peer-reviewed publications
in scientific journals, and 14 invited book chapters and reviews.

Dr. Page describes his tenure as being embedded in neurosurgery
at TMSHMC from 1972 to 2003. During this time, the institution
and he progressed from an exuberant youth to a responsible middle

age and onto the elder's perogative to reminisce. It is the exuberant youth of Hershey that he remembers fondly—those first ten years, when first, George Harrell and then Harry Prystowsky were the Deans. The medical school that George Harrell built was designed to foster clinical and laboratory investigation and collaboration between disciplines. The crescent housed the basic and clinical science departments. The administrative offices were on the concave side of the crescent and each had dedicated laboratories across the hall on the convex side. Neighboring Divisions were situated without regard to the Departments to which they belonged but with regard to common interests. Cross fertilization of ideas was encouraged and the silo mentality was eliminated by design. It was a time when its surgeons were fully integrated into the medical school curriculum and worked side by side with scholars from many disciplines. It was a time when he was privileged to know and work with Richard Bergland (Neurosurgery), Bryce Munger (Anatomy), Howard Morgan (Physiology), Elliot Vesell (Pharmacology), C. Max Lang (Comparative Medicine), Robert Brennan (Neurology), and Robert Greer (Orthopedics) on a variety of projects—laboratory and clinical; a job he described as ideal.

DEPARTMENT of SURGERY, DIVISION of ORTHOPEDIC SURGERY – ROBERT B. GREER, III, M.D., founding Chief (1971-91).

He was born November 28, 1934 in Butler, PA. He graduated from Haverford College (B.A.,1956) and Harvard Medical School (M.D., *cum laude*, 1960).

Greer chose the University of Michigan (1960-61) for his internship in surgery because he was influenced by a young surgeon at Mass General who was going to Michigan to start his career. He had planned to get his board certification in surgery, then pursue a Ph.D., though he was questioning the time required—7 years. However, he changed his career goals when he had an orthopedic rotation. He had hated orthopedic surgery as a medical student because all he did was to hold retractors, but he had a totally different experience at Michigan and made that his focus. His residency was interrupted by the military draft. He was able to secure (Berry Plan) a position at the Walter Reed Army Institute of Research (WRAIR) in the Department of Cellular Physiology. He briefly considered the military as a career until he learned that his options would be very limited. Instead of returning to Michigan to complete his residency, he went to the University of Pittsburgh to assist in his younger brother's care; a hemophiliac with a broken femur. The staff was impressed with him and encouraged him to complete his residency there, and then remain on the faculty, largely because of his mentor, Dr. Henry J. Menkin who was running a research lab studying cartilage. Greer was interested in epiphyseal cartilage; he later assumed Dr Menkin's practice.

Dr Waldhausen (founding Chair of Surgery), whom he did not know, called him to come for a visit. He was quickly recruited because he was fascinated by the opportunity of building a program where nothing had existed before.

His vision/goals were to build a superb clinical program and a strong residency program. Greer had a major role in moving the Elizabethtown Hospital for Crippled Children to TMSHMC.

Greer was a leader in professional societies and journals in his specialty. He published more than 52 scientific articles, two book chapters, and many editorials.

Greer retired relatively early because he had achieved all of his professional goals; citing the Orthopedics Residency Program and children's orthopedics as his major achievements

DEPARTMENT of SURGERY, DIVISION of OTOLARYNGOLOGY-HEAD and NECK SURGERY -- GEORGE H. CONNER, M.D., founding Chief (1973-96).

He was born May 24, 1931 in Evanston, IL. He attended Lake Forest College (IL) receiving a B.A. in 1953. He also received a B.S. from the University of Illinois in 1955. He received the M.D. degree from the University of Illinois in 1957. He completed his internship at St. Luke's Hospital, Chicago, IL (1957-58) and residency in Otolaryngology at the University of Illinois (1958-61). He served as a LCDR, U.S. Navy, Great Lakes Naval Hospital, Chicago, IL (1961-64).

Conner started his academic career as an Instructor of Surgery (Otolaryngology) at the University of Chicago (1964-65), promoted to Assistant Professor (1965-66), and Associate Professor in 1967. He was recruited as Chief, Department of Otolaryngology Henry Ford Hospital and Director, Otological Research Laboratory, Detroit, MI (1967-69). He was subsequently recruited as the Adelot Professor of Otolaryngology and Otolaryngologist-in-Chief, The Johns Hopkins Hospital, Baltimore, MD (1969-70). He returned to Chicago as Associate Attending Otolaryngologist, Rush-Presbyterian- St. Luke's Medical Center (1970-73).

On the basis of these academic affiliations, Conner developed a strong belief that he wanted a fulltime academic, research oriented department, full cooperation between otolaryngologists and plastic surgeons working as a team, and a residency program that would produce academically oriented otolaryngologists in that same mold.

In 1973, Connor was appointed Professor of Surgery and Chief, Division of Otolaryngology-Head and Neck Surgery, The Pennsylvania State University College of Medicine. He began to achieve his dream of an academic research division working as a team with other surgical specialists and residents. Four of his residents went on to become chairs at other institutions.

His research was focused on temporal bone histopathology and disorders of the inner ear. He received many awards/honors for his research and leadership, including the Norvel Pierce Prize (1961), Guest of Honor, Pennsylvania Academy of Otolaryngology Head and Neck Surgery (1994), and Guest of Honor, Eastern Society, The Triological Society (1996). He retired in 1996.

DEPARTMENT of SURGERY, DIVISION of UROLOGY-- THOMAS ROHNER, M.D., founding Chief (1970-2004). He was born January 1, 1936 in Trenton, NJ (died November 22, 2013). He attended Yale University, New Haven, CT (1953-57), receiving a B.A. in 1957. Rohner considered a career as a Presbyterian minister, but chose medicine and attended the University of Pennsylvania School of Medicine, receiving the M.D. degree in 1961.

He did a rotating internship at the Hospital of the University of Pennsylvania, Philadelphia, PA (1961-62) and residencies at the same institution in General Surgery (1962-64), and Urology (1964-67). He then spent 1967-69 as a Major, U.S. Army Medical Corps, 97th General Hospital in Germany and 24th Evacuation Hospital in Vietnam (Berry Plan). After his military service, he returned to the University of Pennsylvania School of Medicine (1969-70), Department of Pharmacology as a USPHS Special Fellow.

Rohner was appointed as an Assistant Professor of Surgery and Chief of the Division of Urology (1970-71), TMSHMC. Waldhausen, Chair of Surgery, was hesitant to appoint him as an Associate Professor because he had not previously had a faculty appointment. However, he was promoted to Associate Professor and Chief (1971-75), and Professor and Chief (1975-2000). He stepped down as Chief of Urology in 2000, but remained as a Professor of Surgery/Urology. He concurrently served as Associate Dean for Clinical Affairs (1996-2000), Chief of Medical Staff (1997-2000), and Senior Vice President, Clinical Operations, all with The Penn State Geisinger Health System. He also served as Interim Chair of Surgery (11/98-8/99).

He served on more than 50 external committees, serving in leadership roles of many; and over 20 internal committees. He was a member of 19 medical society committees, serving in leadership roles of many. His research focused on three major areas: urinary tract smooth muscle; prostate cancer; and urinary incontinence. He is the author/co-author of 18 books and book chapters; and 96 peer-reviewed articles in scientific journals. He received continuous NIH support (1971-85) to support his research programs. He has served as a reviewer for the Journal of Urology since 1989, and Urology since 1993.

CHAPTER 7

ADMINISTRATIVE AND SUPPORT STAFF

ADMINISTRATION – HAROLD (HAL) REINERT
Reinert has had an interesting career. He was born in Slatetown, PA. As a result of a childhood sports injury, he developed osteomyelitis in one of his legs. It never really healed, and he became eligible for a state-funded scholarship. He graduated from Bloomsberg University (B.S). He then taught school for 7 years. He describes that as the best years of his career, but he simply could not raise his family on a teacher's salary.

He responded to an abstract advertisement for salesmen at IBM. At that time, IBM had two divisions; typewriters and punch cards. He was in the latter which became their computer division. Hal was in the top 10% of their salesmen. He sold, and installed, the computer system to the H. B. Reese Candy Company in Hershey, PA. They were so impressed with him, they hired him as a Vice President. However, a few months later, Reese sold the company to the Hershey Chocolate Company, which really offered no opportunity for advancement. He was then offered the position of Controller for The Pennsylvania State University. As part of his orientation for this new position, he was rotated through the various departments to get to know the people, see how they worked, etc. He was assigned to work with Dr Harrell (founding Dean of TMSHMC) who was temporarily assigned to University Park. Reinert's family was still living in Hershey, and he jumped at the chance to return as part of the staff of this new College of Medicine. He never really had an official title, he just did whatever Dr. Harrell wanted him to do. And he did it very well. He developed the offices for the incoming department chairs in a former Hershey student home, hired secretaries and other support staff, and gave talks to many service organizations (on behalf of the Dean) about the new medical school. He had a unique approach to recruiting secretaries. He went to the business departments of the local high schools and said I want the names of your top 3 or 4 students. That became his applicant pool.

Reinert organized, and recruited people for the infrastructure of the medical center; physical plant, personnel, communication services, security, etc. In essence, he functioned as a Business Manager; but he was truly an Assistant to the Dean. He was very bright, and had a very forthright personality. He always did what he thought was best for the medical school.

GRANTS and CONTRACTS -- THURMAN T. GROSSNICKLE, B.S., A.M., Ph.D.,

founding Director, was born July 20, 1924 in his parent's farmhouse near Boonsboro, MD. His father was a farmer, and completed the 8th grade; his mother completed high school and taught elementary school until she married. His parents had different upbringings; his father was a lifelong member of the Church of the Brethren and a lifelong Democrat; his mother was a lifelong member of the Disciples of Christ Church (but was active in her husband's Church) and was a lifelong Republican.

As an only child growing up on the farm, he was involved with daily chores both with animals and housework. He attended Mapleville Elementary School (1930-37) and Boonsboro High School (1937-41). He was active in drama, chorus and newspaper. He attended Bridgewater College, Bridgewater, VA where he was active in drama and glee club as well as working as a Laboratory Assistant (1942-43). He had a military draft deferment during World War II for working on his father's farm. He had leadership positions in the local 4-H club and local and district church activities.

Grossnickle attended Juniata College, Huntington, PA (1947-50 – 3 years). He had completed all of the course requirements by June, 1949 but remained at the college to take additional courses of interest. He was a Research Fellow during Spring, 1950 and was active in drama, speech, chorus, college choir, and chemistry club.

He graduated with a B.S., *cum laude* in 1950 with majors in chemistry and mathematics. He attended Harvard University, Cambridge, MA (1950-52) as a Teaching Fellow (Harvard Teaching Fellowship) and received an A.M. in organic chemistry (1952). During 1952-54, he attended Wayne (State) University, Detroit, MI as a Monsanto Fellow doing research on phenanthrenes and steroids, resulting in 5 scientific publications. He received the Ph.D. degree in organic chemistry in 1955.

He attended the University of Rochester, Rochester, NY (1954-56) as a Postdoctoral Fellow doing research on alkaloids and natural products. In 1956, he accepted a position at Bridgewater College as Assistant Professor of Chemistry (1956-59; promoted to Associate Professor 1959-61) with a full teaching load in chemistry; and conducting organic chemistry research with grant support from the National Institutes of Health, the National Science Foundation, and the Research Corporation.

Grossnickle joined the National Institutes of Health (NIH), first as a Research Grants Officer in the National Institute of Arthritis and Metabolic Diseases (1961-63), then as Urology Program Director (1963-64). He transferred to the Division of Research Grants as Executive Secretary, Medicinal Chemistry B Study Section (1964-72).

Although he had an enjoyable and productive career at the NIH, he and his wife were not satisfied with the living conditions in that area. They had 4 small children and chose a neighborhood in close proximity to a good school. However, they noticed almost every week ambulances were going to the school. The problem was drug abuse. They decided that they would have to move. They spent several weekends traveling through MD and surrounding states looking for a place that he could work and a more suitable community in which to raise a family. Another requirement was in proximity to a Church of the Brethren and large enough to have a strong youth program. On one such trip, they were impressed with Central Pennsylvania, and he stopped at TMSHMC to inquire about possible employment. It was fortuitous that Waldhausen, as Interim Dean, had just received permission from the University President to hire someone to direct the Office of Grants and Contracts. All grants and contracts had previously been processed by the Office of Sponsored Programs at University Park, a very cumbersome arrangement.

Grossnickle was hired in 1972 as Assistant Provost of Grants and Contracts. He was promoted to Director of Grants and Contracts in 1974, apparently after proving to the University that he was competent to do the job.

He was very meticulous; he was very familiar with the NIH procedures, and his scientific background added to his creditability. He was well known for his "purple pen"; he used purple ink to highlight errors and for suggestions that he thought would be helpful in achieving success in funding. He was not at all dictatorial but really meant to be helpful, although not all faculty appreciated his efforts on their behalf. However, he did raise the bar for excellence, which was a factor in our success. Another thing that some faculty did not like was that he processed all grants and contracts in the order that they were received; he gave no special favors for tardiness. He ran his office with efficiency. He only had one professional assistant and one secretary.

Grossnickle retired in 1990, devoting his life to his church, and various charitable organizations.

HOSPITAL ADMINISTRATION—JOHN A. RUSSELL, M.H.A., FACHE – First Director of the Teaching Hospital of The Milton S. Hershey Medical Center (1967-75).

Russell was born in Flint, MI, grew up in Michigan and went to college at Western Michigan (B.S., 1954). He had joined the Army ROTC to help finance his college education, and was obligated to enter the Army. Although he was trained in the Quartermaster Corps, he was assigned to the Medical Corps, and spent two years in Germany running a military hospital. Some of the physicians assigned to that hospital encouraged him to return to school and study Hospital Administration. He did so after his discharge, receiving the M.H.A. (1958) from the University of Michigan. It was a two year program with the second year as an internship. He did his internship at the Evanston Hospital which is affiliated with Northwestern University. After completing his degree, he was asked to remain at Evanston where he served as Administrative Resident, Administrative Assistant, and Assistant Administrator (1957-60). A former Professor at the University of Michigan was recruited to be the hospital director at the University of Wisconsin, and asked Russell to join him as Assistant Superintendent, and then Associate Superintendent and Chief Operating Officer at the University of Wisconsin Medical Center Hospital (1961-67). His administrative duties included operational responsibility for nearly all phases. He also coordinated all aspects of a major planning and development project to relocate the University Hospital to a new site.

Dr George T. Harrell, founding Dean, TMSHMC asked him to come to Hershey to see if he would be interested in the position of Hospital Director. He came three times before making a decision. The hospital consisted of architectural drawings at that time. He accepted the challenge, primarily because of his confidence in Dr. Harrell and his vision. He oversaw the final internal plans and recruited staff for the heads of 32 hospital departments. It was through his efforts that we were able to build, and open, a modern hospital that became financially stable within two years.

Russell left in 1975 to become the Senior Vice President of The Hospital Association of Pennsylvania. In 1983, he became the President of that organization, and served in that capacity until 1998. From 1995 to 1998, he also served as President of the Institute for Healthy Communities. Since that time, he has remained active as a Consultant in Health Care Management, and Professor of Practice in the Penn State Health Care Administration Graduate Program.

HOSPITAL ADMINISTRATION – WILLIAM E. CORLEY,

B.A., M.H.A. – second director of the Teaching Hospital of The Milton S. Hershey Medical Center (1975-78)

Corley was born and raised in Pittsburgh, PA. He excelled as an athlete (football, basketball, track) in high school and college. He received his B.A. (1964) from William and Mary, Williamsburg, VA, and his M.H.A from Duke University (1966).

He started his professional career as an administrative assistant at Duke University. He then entered the U.S. Army to fulfill his Army ROTC obligation. He was initially assigned to the Armed Forces Institute of Pathology/Walter Reed Army Medical Center. After a year he volunteered to serve in Viet Nam. After his military service he worked for a large consulting firm, Booz, Allen &Hamilton. He played a role in developing health care programs in Canada. Although he enjoyed his work, the travel required by the job led him to be the Associate Hospital Director at the Chandler Medical Center, University of KY (1971-75). In 1975 he was named Hospital Director of TMSHMC.

Upon his appointment at Hershey, he quickly realized that the hospital had significant financial difficulties and a weak infrastructure. Corley recruited talented people and corrected most problems. He recognized the need for a collaborative network (NOT a merger) of hospitals for greater operational efficiency and improved patient care. He believed that this would surely be the future of medical care in the U.S. Unfortunately, the leadership did not concur with his plan to develop a network of hospitals, and he left to become a Hospital Director in Ohio. After six years as the President and CEO at the Akron General Medical Center, he became the CEO of Community Health Network in Indianapolis, IN, a healthcare system with six hospitals. He has received several awards, including the highest honor bestowed on individuals by the Indiana Governor; and served on many boards.

HOSPITAL ADMINISTRATION – J. KNOX SINGLETON, B.S., M.H.A.

Singleton was born in NC in 1948, and moved to Murphy, N.C. shortly thereafter. He started his post-secondary education at Maryville College, then transferred to the University of North Carolina where he earned a B.S. in Business Administration in 1970, *Phi Beta Kappa*. He received his Master's Degree in Health Administration from Duke University in 1973. He then accepted a Fellowship at Guy's Hospital in London, England. He chose this fellowship because he thought many aspects of the English health system would emerge in the U.S.

He was recruited as Assistant Director of the Teaching Hospital of TMSHMC in 1975, and promoted to Director (1978-83), during a period of substantial growth and development of the medical center. He was impressed with the relative young age of the various leaders, their collegiality, and vision for success.

Singleton was then recruited, in 1983, as the COO of Inova Health System, and soon became the CEO. Inova is one of the nation's most integrated and most wired health care delivery systems, and one of the largest in the metropolitan Washington, D.C. region. He is very active in a variety of community organizations. He has received many awards for these activities, including honorary degrees from the North Virginia Community College and Cumberland College in Williamsburg, VA.

HOSPITAL ADMINISTRATION -- HOWARD J. PETERSON, B.S., M.H.A., Executive Director, University Hospital (1983-89)

Peterson was born and raised in Owatonna, MN. He started his post-secondary education at the General Motors Institute which was oriented towards Industrial Administration. After one year he transferred to the University of Minnesota where he had three minors but no major. His original thoughts were to go to graduate school in some field. When he was a junior and reviewing graduate program brochures, he came across the brochure for the Hospital

Administration program at Minnesota. He re-arranged his courses and worked as a nursing assistant at the University of Minnesota to learn more about patient care. Finalizing his career goal, he enrolled in the graduate program in Hospital Administration. During his residency training he decided that he wanted to be in academic, as opposed to community, hospital administration.

After graduation, he went to the University of Michigan as an assistant to the Senior Vice President for Operations. He was given considerable latitude, and gained experience in team management of hospital administration.

Peterson was recruited to TMSHMC in 1983. As part of his recruitment, he requested that the name be changed from Teaching Hospital to University Hospital, in part, because he believed that a name change was important to better reflect its mission and goals. A particular goal was to better integrate nursing into a higher level of leadership and patient care. He considered himself to be relatively young and inexperienced for his role. However, he surrounded himself with competent people, and gave them the authority to do their job. He also relied heavily on physicians to ensure compatibility between administration and patient care.

Peterson had a keen insight on the roles of academic and community health centers. Academic centers should be at the forefront of innovative and scholarly research as well as the handling of complex patient cases. Community hospitals should benefit from this new information in providing high quality patient care.

He is currently a Partner of TRG Healthcare, LLC and Brightworks Management, LLC

HOSPITAL ADMINISTRATION – JOHN E. MAY, III

May was born and raised in Mississippi. He had an interest in science and majored in biology at the University of Mississippi. Still undecided about his career, he decided to teach. He taught science to junior and senior students in central FL. One day, he scheduled a Career Day for his students. One of the presenters was from a small university in the area. It was there that he learned they had a degree program in Medical Records, something that he did not know even existed. He pursued that goal and graduated.

His first job in hospital administration was in central TN. After a few years, he was looking for opportunities to advance and saw an advertisement for a position at TMSHMC. He was appointed Manager, Medical Records and Administrative Assistant in 1976. He quickly assumed the responsibility for Utilization Review and Quality Assurance program. Mays took advantage of working in other hospital administration areas. In the ensuing years he served as Assistant Hospital Director (1979-83), Acting Hospital Director (1983), Director, Outpatient and Emergency Operations (1984-90), Senior Associate Director, University Hospitals (1991-96), Hospital Director (1997), Vice President, Administrative Associate, Medicine, Penn State Geisinger Health System (1997-2000), Interim Chief Operating Officer (2000-02), and Chief Compliance Officer (2002-2010). His cooperative spirit, commitment to excellence, and job knowledge made him a valued team member.

PERSONNEL -- Nicholas Otzel, B. S. was born February 5, 1942 in Harrisburg, PA. He attended Mount Saint Mary's College, Emmitsburg, MD and received a B.S. in Business Administration with a major in Economics and a minor in Accounting in 1965. He worked as an Underwriter for the Nationwide Insurance Company, Harrisburg, PA 1965-68. During this time he received a Commercial Pilot license with multi engine and instrument ratings, and worked as a corporate pilot for Capitol Products, Mechanicsburg, PA (1968-70). He enjoyed flying and would have preferred flying commercial aircraft; however, he could not meet the height requirement. He then worked for the Commonwealth of PA, Department of Revenue, Harrisburg, PA, computing the tax of firms with less than $200,000 valuation that transact business in PA (1970-71).

Otzel was hired as an Administrative Assistant by the Department of Surgery (1971-73). He then became a Personnel Assistant in the Department of Personnel Services (1973-75), promoted to Personnel Officer (1975-81), Director of Personnel (1981-85), Associate

Director of Human Resources (1985-88). He became Director of Administration, Department of Family and Community Medicine (1988-97). He was named Manager of Human Resources, Office of the Controller in 1997 until his retirement in 2002.

He had the perfect combination of traits for personnel/human resources: knowledgeable, including who to contact for answers; extremely conscientious in making sure that everyone was treated fairly and compassionately. His only fault was the feeling that perhaps he didn't have all the answers or did not give someone the correct information; quite frankly, no one could have done better.

EPILOGUE

Twenty-eight years have now elapsed since the period covered by this historical collection (1967-87); and 6 years since we began to assemble data. As stated earlier, it was believed that a lapse of 25 years was appropriate, and necessary, before making an assessment of results. However, some interviewees elected to comment on events beyond this time frame. We have retained those comments in their edited, conversational English interviews. As will be noted in reading the edited transcripts, it was somewhat surprising about the occasional misperceptions of events even after 25 years.

It was noted that Presidents choose their Deans, Deans choose their Chairs and Chairs choose their faculty. This, for the most part, has remained true. Leadership has, for the most part, been quite variable at all levels. Search committees have been established for all three levels of leadership but, in essence, they have had little impact on the final selection. This suggests that Search Committees have little function except to help select candidates and provide information to candidates.

There was very little turnover in the Chairs during the first 30 years, reflecting the Founding Dean Harrell's desire to select promising candidates who would achieve their potential here and not use it as a stepping stone to go elsewhere. This was very evident in the national and international recognition of most of the early founders.

The interviewees expressed the opinion that, generally, successors of the Founders were not up to the same caliber. However, these beliefs may have been skewed somewhat by comparing new appointees at the beginning of their administrative career with those that had matured and retired. By and large, the first group of Founding Chairs did achieve national, and international, recognition. Their successors may eventually achieve these same accolades, but the trajectory does not yet seem promising; several interviewees describe many of them as "caretakers" or "managers" rather than leaders capable of taking us to the next level.

Presidents and Deans seem to be in their own class, operating individually, whereas Chairs tend to succeed in close and cooperative concert with their faculty. Founding Chairs had the advantage of choosing their own faculty, whereas their successors inherited most of their senior faculty; almost a step family arrangement. Even though they may have bargained for a few additional faculty appointments, integration of the new family and loyalties is always difficult.

Funding has continued to be a challenge. One main reason is that, as an institution, we are essentially self-supporting with minimal state support. Patient care income has dramatically improved, but other sources of funding have become more of a problem, especially in research, most noticeable in the basic sciences. Availability of research funds has diminished over time. In 1967, the institution had approximately $27 million ($192 million in 2014 adjusted for inflation) direct research costs, primarily from the NIH. The perception is that our funding has fallen relatively (in 2014 it was about $87 million including clinical trials). However, a better measure might be our ranking of NIH funding. It is easy to point to the decrease in NIH direct funding; however, an increasing amount of the overall NIH funds is being diverted to indirect costs (Facilities and Administration)—especially for regulatory activities. This is a national problem of great concern. One also has to look at the number and amounts of research grants being submitted.

Also, the question arises: how we define research? Among the Founders, there was almost universal belief that research was essential for good teaching and patient care, i.e. the acquisition and dissemination of new information and its application. There is no question that funded investigators are doing that plus keeping up to date in their field. Others are mainly disseminating second hand information.

This questions the quality of institutional leadership. It is true that there are many detractors, e. g., continual changes in the medical school curriculum, a perceived lack of focus on education, and an increasing emphasis on the "bottom line." There is no question of the importance of financial stability, but one can question the overall balance between education/research/patient care versus operational income.

We, the Founders, were very fortunate in our beginning, having a sense of future challenges, collegiality, scholarship and minimal restraints. There are still few constraints, but the collegiality and scholarship are not as evident as they were in the levels of leadership. There seems to be much reduced interpersonal communication as space in the institution greatly expanded. People are hard to locate to discuss issues and to achieve problem solving. Our interpersonal communications need to be improved and facilitated.

Space has always been a problem. In the beginning, we had too much space because we had a small faculty and a building that was designed for growth. Early faculty were assigned two laboratories rather than leave space unoccupied. As the faculty grew, they had to relinquish space. Continued growth resulted in more concessions. More than one Dean has commented that space is more of an emotional issue than salaries, since salaries of colleagues is not generally known, whereas space is easily visualized; sometimes down to as little difference as one foot. Space needs change significantly with time due to technology advancements. This is further complicated by the accumulation of outdated reagents and unused equipment. There is a widely held belief that almost any institution could achieve at least 25% additional laboratory space merely by removing outdated reagents and unused equipment. However, this requires strong, and knowledgeable, leadership at the college and department level.

There have been attempts to address space allocations, but with many failures. In reality, every space decision makes someone happy, and someone mad. Ultimate success will probably only be achieved by giving each department/unit definitive, "sacred" space to meet their core needs, space for new investigators, and space for investigators between funding (for a reasonable period of time). This is essential to give faculty and chairs a sense of ownership. Additional space should be flexible and based solely on funding and productivity, with the full anticipation that there will be changes in its occupants.

Space is often reduced in effectiveness when investigators want to design their "own" space. Unless they are trained in architecture/ engineering, few are able to conceptualize space. This is further compromised when walls are moved without a concomitant re-design of the HVAC support.

The Milton S. Hershey Medical Center has demonstrated many significant strengths. These include scholarship and leadership locally, nationally, and internationally; research discoveries; training and development of students, residents, fellows, and young faculty; and the care and treatment of patients to a new level. If we achieve the positive aspects of this trajectory through the next segments of our history, then we will continue to realize "The Impossible Dream".

APPENDICES

Appendices are available at ScholarSphere, a service that was collaboratively developed by two units at Penn State: the University Libraries and Information Technology Services. Please access per directions as follows:

Select from the four (4) Appendices

1. Enter the selected URL into the address box/location bar (NOT the "search box") located at the top of your internet browser and press the "Enter" key to access ScholarSphere.

2. Review the list of available files to identify which document you want to review (the list may continue on the next screen(s) – the number of items per screen can be changed from the Drop-down menu right above the list).

3. To open a particular file, go to the "Action" column on the right. Click on the arrow in the corresponding "Select an action" box, and then click "Download File". The full document may then open on your screen.
4. If the document does not open, you will see a document icon on the bottom left of your screen. Click on the document icon to open the file.

Appendix 1. Curriculum Vitae (as of the time of the interview) of 62 Founders. For the book, we were able to interview 55 of the 62.

https://scholarsphere.psu.edu/collections/5712mh50f

Abt, Arthur, Department of Pathology

Bardin, Wayne, Department of Medicine, Division of Endocrinology (3 files)

Berlin, Cheston, Department of Pediatrics

Biebuyck, Julien, Department of Anesthesia

Bryant, Fred, Library

Burnside, John, Department of Medicine

Conner, George, Department of Surgery

Corley, William, Hospital Administration

Davidson, Eugene, Department of Biological Chemistry

Demers, Laurence, Department of Pathology

DeMuth, William, Department of Surgery

Dossett, John, Department of Pediatrics

Egeland, Janice, Department of Behavioral Science

Eyster, Elaine, Department of Medicine

Gault, James, Department of Medicine

Glaser, Ronald, Department of Microbiology

Greer, Robert, Department of Surgery

Grossnickle, Thurman T, Administration, Grants and Contracts

Houts, Peter, Department of Behavioral Science

Jefferson, Leonard, Department of Physiology

Jeffries, Graham, Department of Medicine (2 files)

Jenkins, David, Jr, Department of Medicine

Kales, Anthony, Department of Psychiatry

Krieg, Arthur, Department of Pathology

Ladda, Roger, Department of Pediatrics

Lang, C. Max, Department of Comparative Medicine

Leaman, David, Department of Medicine

Leaman, Thomas, Department of Family & Community Medicine

Lehman, Lois, Library

Lipton, Allan, Department of Medicine

Maisels, M. Jeffrey, Department of Pediatrics

May, John, Hospital Administration

Miller, Kenneth, Department of Radiology
Morgan, Howard E., Department of Physiology
Mortel, Rodrique, Department of Obstetrics & Gynecology
Muller, Arnold, Department of Medicine
Munger, Bryce, Department of Anatomy
Naeye, Richard, Department of Pathology
Nahrwold, David, Department of Surgery
Nelson, Nicholas, Department of Pediatrics
Otzel, Nicholas, Administration
Page, Robert, Department of Surgery
Pattishall, Evan G., Department of Behavioral Science
Pegg, Anthony, Department of Physiology
Peterson, Howard, Hospital Administration
Pierce, William, Department of Surgery
Rapp, Fred, Department of Microbiology
Rohner, Thomas, Department of Surgery
Rohrer, G. Victor, Department of Radiology
Russell, John, Hospital Administration
Santen, Richard, Department of Medicine
Severs, Walter, Department of Pharmacology
Singleton, Knox, Hospital Administration
Stenger, Vincent, Department of Obstetrics & Gynecology
Vastyan, Al, Department of Humanities
Vesell, Elliot, Department of Pharmacology
Waldhausen, John, Department of Surgery
Wassner, Steven, Department of Pediatrics
Weidner, William, Department of Radiology
Yeakel, Allen, Department of Anesthesiology
Zagon, Ian, Department of Anatomy
Zelis, Robert, Department of Medicine (2 files)

Appendix 2. Transcripts of Interviews

https://scholarsphere.psu.edu/collections/x346dk56t

Abt, Arthur, Department of Pathology

Bardin, Wayne, Department of Medicine

Berlin, Cheston, Department of Pediatrics

Biebuyck, Julien, Department of Anesthesia

Burnside, John, Department of Medicine

Conner, George, Department of Surgery

Corley, William, Hospital Administration

Davidson, Eugene, Department of Biological Chemistry

Demers, Laurence, Department of Pathology

DeMuth, William, Department of Surgery

Dossett, John, Department of Pediatrics

Egeland, Janice, Department of Behavioral Science

Eyster, M. Elaine, Department of Medicine

Gault, James, Department of Medicine

Glaser, Ronald, Department of Microbiology

Greer, Robert, Department of Surgery

Grossnickle, Thurman T., Administration, Grants & Contracts

Houts, Peter, Department of Behavioral Sciences

Jefferson, Leonard, Department of Physiology

Jeffries, Graham, Department of Medicine

Jenkins, David Jr, Department of Medicine

Krieg, Arthur, Department of Pathology

Ladda, Roger, Department of Pediatrics

Lang, C. Max, Department of Comparative Medicine

Leaman, David, Department of Medicine

Leaman, Thomas, Department of Family & Community Medicine

Lipton, Allan, Department of Medicine

Maisels, Jeffrey, Department of Pediatrics

May, John, Hospital Administration

Miller, Kenneth, Department of Radiology

Mortel, Rodrique, Department of Obstetrics & Gynecology

Muller, Arnold, Department of Medicine

Munger, Bryce, Department of Anatomy

Naeye, Richard, Department of Pathology

Nahrwold, David, Department of Surgery

Nelson, Nicholas, Department of Pediatrics

Otzel, Nicholas, Administration

Page, Robert, Department of Surgery

Pegg, Anthony, Department of Physiology

Peterson, Howard, Hospital Administration

Pierce, William, Department of Surgery

Reinert, Harold, Administration

Rohner, Thomas, Department of Surgery

Rohrer, G. Victor, Department of Radiology

Russell, John, Hospital Administration

Santen, Richard, Department of Medicine

Severs, Walter, Department of Pharmacology

Singleton, Knox, Hospital Administration

Stenger, Vincent, Department of Obstetrics & Gynecology

Vastyan, Al, Department of Humanities

Vesell, Elliot, Department of Pharmacology

Waldhausen, John, Department of Surgery

Wassner, Steven, Department of Pediatrics

Yeakel, Allen, Department of Anesthesiology

Zelis, Robert, Department of Medicine

Appendix 3. References and Supplemental Materials

https://scholarsphere.psu.edu/collections/x346dk573

Biebuyck. Anesthesiology Department Lecture (10/9/10)
Jeffries. 1st 22 Years
Miller
     Elmer and the Gray Fox
     A Health Physicist Laments
     A Raccoon in the Chimney
Page. Embedded in Neurosurgery
Vesell. Recollections of the Inception of the Department of Pharmacology in 1968
     at Penn State College of Medicine
Waldhausen. The Early Years at Penn State/Hershey: Reflections of a Surgeon
Yeakel. Joseph Priestley Lecture: History of the Penn State University Department
     of Anesthesiology
Historical Research Space and Research Funding
     Gross Square Feet by Laboratory (Research)/Office/Education: 1967/!987/2015
     Campus Map

Other References (not on URL)
Berlin, C. M. Ideas, Collaboration, and Replication
     J. Pharmacol. Ther. 2007 Vol 12:16-22
Lang, C. M. The Cost of Animal Research. LAB ANIMAL, Vol 38, Number
     10, October, 2009
Miller, K., Groff,L., Erdman, M., and King, S. Lessons Learned in Preparing
     for Receipt of Large Numbers of Contaminated Individuals. Health Physics
     89:2, S42-47, August 2005

Other References (Available for sale from the publisher)
*Planning Medical Center Facilities for Education, Research, and Public Service.
     George T. Harrell, 1974, The Pennsylvania State University Press, University
     Park, PA

*The Impossible Dream: The Founding of The Milton S. Hershey Medical Center, C. Max Lang, 2010, Authorhouse, 1633 Liberty Drive, Bloomington. IN. www. authorhouse.com

*Elmer and Me, Kenneth L. Miller, 2011. Authorhouse, 1633 Liberty Drive, Bloomington, IN www.authorhouse.com

*I Am From Haiti, Rodrique Mortel, 2000. The Mortel Family Foundation, P.O. Box 405, Hershey, PA 17033, mortel@mortelfoundation.org

*Finding a Home in a World at War, 1929-1963: John A. Waldhausen, 2005. Gateway Press, Inc, 3600 Clipper Mill Rd, Suite 260, Baltimore, MD, www. gatewaypress.com

Appendix 4. Background material for *The Impossible Dream*

https://scholarsphere.psu.edu/collections/x346dk55j

PLEASE NOTE: The following materials were used as background for *The Impossible Dream, The Founding of The Milton S. Hershey Medical Center of The Pennsylvania State University* (C. Max Lang, Editor, 2010, Authorhouse, 1633 Liberty Drive, Bloomington, IN 47403, www.authorhouse.com), and partially referenced in this book. Because the material was so large, it was decided to condense it into the text. Most of the material has not previously been made available to the general public. Individual copies may be made for personal use, but PLEASE DO NOT DUPLICATE FOR FURTHER DISTRIBUTION WITHOUT PERMISSION from the editor.

File	Contents
TID 1	Background Information
	The Impossible Dream
	Congressional Record-U.S. House of Representatives (August 27, 1963)
	Lebanon Daily News (February 6, 1964)
	Hershey Hospital (4/14/65)
	Presentation/Request
	Summary of Meeting
	Salaries
	Pictures (circa 1966)
	Gro-Mor Barn
	Typical chairman's office in Long Lane
TID 2	William Christensen (Construction Supervisor) Interview
	Letter of invitation
	Curriculum Vitae
	Cost of Building
	Letter from Wilkinson to Shoemaker
	Pictures (circa 1964-67)
	Construction site (circa 1964)

Construction site (circa 1964)

Groundbreaking (February 26, 1966)

Groundbreaking (February 26, 1966)

Construction of Basic Science Wing (1966) and Clinical Science
Wing (1968)

Construction of the tunnel (1967)

The "Great Fire" on the 5th floor of the Basic Science Wing and
aftermath

TID 3   George T. Harrell, Jr. (Founding Dean) Interview

Picture

Curriculum Vitae

Letter of Invitation

The Dean Search

TID 4   John O. Hershey (Hershey Trust Co & Milton S. Hershey School)
Interview

Letter of Invitation

Picture

Curriculum Vitae

Suggestions from Hershey Estates

TID 5   Samuel F. Hinkle (Pres, Hershey Chocolate Co & Hershey Trust)

Letter of Recollections (6/10/71)

TID 6   C. Max Lang, first faculty appointment

Self interview

Curriculum Vitae

The Early Years – Commitment

Site pictures

TID 7   Harold S. Mohler (Pres, Hershey Chocolate Co & Hershey Trust)
Interview

Picture

Curriculum Vitae

TID 8   Gilbert Nurick (Lawyer) Interview
                Letter of Invitation
                Curriculum Vitae
                Picture

TID 9   Eric Walker (President, TPSU) Interview
                Letter of Invitation
                Picture
                Curriculum Vitae
                Memos to File
                Carpenter Situation/Advisory Committee

TID 10   Arthur Whiteman (Pres, Hershey Bank & Hershey Trust Co) Interview
                Letter of Invitation
                Curriculum Vitae
                Presentations

TID 11   Legal Proceedings
                May 8, 1963 Factual Statement (as delivered to the Attorney General of the Commonwealth of Pennsylvania) Dictionary definition of *Cy Pres*
                July 19, 1963 Petition for *Cy Pres* award
                Aug 23, 1963 Memorandum (background for the *Cy Pres* petition
                Aug 23, 1963 Decree for transferring funds to establish The Milton S. Hershey Medical Center
                Aug 27, 1963 Affiliation Agreement between the M. S. Hershey Foundation and The Pennsylvania State University
                Nov, 1968 Memorandum (petition for modification to substitute The Pennsylvania State University as successor trustee to the M. S. Foundation for The Milton S. Hershey Medical Center
                Dec 17, 1968 Decree approving The Pennsylvania State University as Successor Trustee

Printed in the United States
By Bookmasters